Behavior of the Fetus

Behavior of the Fetus

William P. Smotherman

Department of Psychology
State University of New York at Binghamton
Binghamton, New York

Scott R. Robinson

Department of Zoology
Oregon State University
Corvallis, Oregon

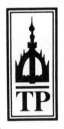

THE TELFORD PRESS
Caldwell, New Jersey

THE TELFORD PRESS, INC.
285 Bloomfield Avenue, Caldwell, New Jersey, 07006

Library of Congress Cataloging-in-Publication Data

Behavior of the fetus.

Includes bibliographies and index.
1. Fetus. 2. Prenatal influence. 3. Fetus—Growth.
4. Maternal-fetal exchange. 5. Neuropsychology.
I. Smotherman, William P. II. Robinson, Scott R.,
1952–   . [DNLM: 1. Behavior. 2. Fetus.
WQ 210 B419]
RG613.B44   1988   612'.647   88–16071
ISBN 0–936923–13–X
ISBN 0–936923–14–8 (pbk.)

Dedication

To William and Margaret Smotherman, who were attentive to the details of my early development.

WPS

And to Karen (she knows why).

SRR

Table of Contents

Preface

This decade has seen a resurgence of interest in the prenatal development of behavior in mammals. In part, the rediscovery of the fetus has been promoted by new medical technology that permits noninvasive, indirect monitoring of fetal activity, such as real-time ultrasonography. At the same time, researchers working with nonhuman animals have improved surgical procedures and other experimental techniques that permit direct observation of fetal behavior. Together, indirect monitoring of human fetuses and direct observation and experimentation with nonhuman fetuses are replacing speculations of the past with empirical data about prenatal life and its role in the ontogeny of behavior.

Medical, ethical and social issues also underscore the need for understanding fetal behavior. Abnormal fetal activity has been implicated in the etiology of certain forms of congenital birth defect. Prospective parents want to know what life is like for the unborn child and how they might influence its prenatal development. Of course, ethical and technological considerations limit what can be learned about the human fetus, so researchers utilize animal models to begin to assess the abilities of the fetus before birth and the importance of prenatal behavior and intrauterine environment on subsequent postnatal development.

This volume provides a summary of the current state of thought in the field of prenatal behavioral research. Historically, researchers have approached the study of the embryo and fetus from many different fields of inquiry, ranging from child development, pediatric medicine and obstetrics to behavioral embryology, neurobiology and psychobiology. Technical reports are dispersed across many scholarly journals that often do not share a common audience. This volume attempts to unite these diverse interests by providing a concise introduction to major conceptual issues, theoretical questions and empirically-derived speculations as framed by leading scholars in the field of prenatal behavioral research.

Concepts and Issues

On the Nature and Function of Prenatal Behavior

Myron A. Hofer
Department of Developmental Psychobiology
New York State Psychiatric Institute
Columbia University
New York, New York

Customarily, we date the beginnings of our life by our birth, as if the previous nine months of our existence never occurred or were lived out in a form that bore no relationship to the rest of our life history. Embryologists, who have long been interested in this period of development, continue the pattern of selective inattention by ignoring one of the most striking characteristics of embryos of all species—their behavior. Although there have been a number of notable exceptions, starting with Wilhelm Preyer in 1885, embryologists generally have focused their attention entirely on the remarkable changes in form prior to birth or hatching while ignoring function. A sampling of the many embryological texts available today reveals that the vast majority do not even inform their readers that embryos start to show frequent and patterned movements at a remarkably early stage, although this fact has been known for generations. Developmental psychologists support this silence very effectively by beginning their accounts of behavior development with the newborn period, 7 months after overt behavior has begun to occur. In the absence of systematic scientific attention, theories and even advice on prenatal behavior have derived from the imagination of the curious.

There are a number of recent events that are rapidly changing our attitudes toward the 'terra incognita' of prenatal behavior: (a) the increasing survival of very early preterm infants who force us to confront directly this period of our lives; (b) technological advances in embryo transplantation and artificial insemination which date our beginnings in as clear a fashion as the event of birth, but nine months earlier; (c) the invention of high resolution ultrasound recording which is allowing us to study human fetal behavior for the first time with precision and safety; (d) the rapid advances in developmental neuroscience which are revealing the existence and importance of very early neural function during the embryonic period; (e) the emergence of new concepts of development which allow us to understand the adaptive value of prenatal behavior by integrating

3

structural and functional processes, and by considering intrauterine and postnatal events as parts of a coherent system established by evolution.

The task of understanding postnatal behavior development has been greatly impeded by our ignorance about the origins of behavior and about the nature of the intrauterine period in general. It is like trying to build a house without a foundation, and therefore we need to approach the subject of prenatal behavior with the intent of exploring how recent developments in the field are beginning to provide such a foundation. The research findings reported in the various chapters of this book quite literally illuminate a new landscape. And the nature of what they reveal about the intrauterine period of development and of prenatal behavior is particularly interesting because it is so puzzling. Our difficulty in answering simple questions illustrates our conceptual ignorance. What exactly are the developmental roles of the special environmental conditions we encounter during the prenatal period? What is the purpose of our advanced sensorimotor capabilities and our incessant activity throughout most of this period?

ONTOGENETIC ADAPTATION

Current views of psychological development emphasize continuity and progression. Where different stages clearly exist, the role of each as preparation for a subsequent stage is stressed. The discovery that mammalian embryos begin to move very early in the prenatal period and that sensory systems also become functional long before they are needed, has caused us to attempt to extend the same developmental view back into the intrauterine period: if sensorimotor function is present before birth, the fetus must be practicing or preparing in some way for the behavioral tasks of the postnatal environment. And indeed, examples can be found which seem to fit this point of view. But to most informed scientists the major portion of 'precocious' sensorimotor development is difficult to explain in these terms. The recent appearance of "fetal universities" in some communities dramatizes the absurdities to which the 'progressive' view of behavior development can be taken.

The bias in our thinking is exemplified by the tendency for behavioral scientists, even in the developmental area, to forget or misremember the answer to a simple question about our early development: who produces the placenta and membranes? It is disconcerting for us to realize that it is the fetus and not the mother who develops these large, complex structures and then discards them at birth. It makes our developmental plan seem more like that of the tadpole and the frog than is comfortable for us. The useful idea stemming from this little-appreciated fact about our origins is that the intrauterine period of our life involves a very different set of physical adaptations from the postnatal period and that the forms and functions of behavior also are likely to be substantially different in the two periods of our life.

The evolutionary path of the placental mammals has maximized the elements of protection and of control of their progeny, with a constant nutrient supply being provided to a few relatively large offspring. This path diverged from the plan of earlier vertebrates, which relied upon many, smaller offspring, each provided with nutrient yolk sufficient for independent development until self-feeding. The mammalian strategy, however, retained some of the elements of the larval specializations so characteristic of earlier vertebrates (as represented by the tadpole stage of today's amphibians). The general developmental principle involved has been termed "ontogenetic adaptation" by Oppenheim (1981). This term refers to the observation that early stages of development, which predictably involve different environments from those of later stages, evolve "specific morphological, biochemical, physiological and behavioral mechanisms which are different from the adult and which may require modification, suppression or even destruction before the adult stage can be obtained." The formation and subsequent shedding of the placenta at birth is a familiar example of a specific morphological mechanism of this sort. This paper will consider a number of behavioral mechanisms which can be understood in terms of the concept of ontogenetic adaptation.

As adults, we tend to have a parochial view of development and must keep reminding ourselves that it is the whole developmental plan that is selected by evolution, not simply adult traits. Thus, selective pressures operate at all stages of development and the immediate adaptive advantage conferred by a behavior, or any other function, acting in the predictable environment of a particular developmental stage, contributes as much to its selection, as does its role as a building block for the adult trait. Thus, a trait which promotes increased efficiency of survival only in an early phase of development will be selected as readily as an adult trait which accounts directly for increased reproductive fitness (Oyama, 1985; Raff & Kaufman, 1983).

A recent discovery in postnatal behavior development will illustrate this point. It was long assumed that nursing in mammals was a precursor of independent feeding, a kind of imperfect form of the adult behavior pattern. This led to the belief that an infant must suckle in order to eat, as it was also believed it must crawl in order to walk. This sequential, progressive view of development has been applied to almost every aspect of psychological development by the major figures of this century. However, we know that suckling and crawling experience are not at all necessary for the later appearance of eating and walking behavior (Hall & Williams, 1983; see Thelen, this volume). Hall (1975) found that independent feeding developed on time and entirely normally in juvenile rats that were raised artificially and never suckled. The controls for independent feeding are different in major ways from those for suckling and they develop coincidentally with suckling rather than sequentially. Suckling thus is an example of an ontogenetic adaptation in the rat, and is better understood in terms of its function during the pre-weaning period of development than in terms of its role as a precursor of the later independent feeding of juvenile and adult stages. The fact that all infant mammals give up nursing behavior, but not feeding behavior, indicates how development is discontinuous and how certain behavioral processes regress or are eliminated (like the placenta and membranes) while vital functions continue to be carried out.

In summary then, evolution selects a whole historical process, some elements of which are necessary only for a given period and its unique conditions, while other elements serve primarily as building blocks for subsequent stages, having little other function in earlier stages of development. Naturally, many processes share in both these attributes. The concept of ontogenetic adaptation can be useful to organize and understand many of the special features of the intrauterine period, as well as some of the features of subsequent development. It can unify our view of development from prenatal to postnatal periods (see Smotherman & Robinson, this volume) as well as do traditional themes of epigenetic progression, and adds considerable explanatory power. Since the two themes are not incompatible, they can be taken together and as such give us a useful concept of development with which to approach the papers in this volume that discuss the special properties of intrauterine life.

THE INTRAUTERINE ENVIRONMENT

One of the limitations of the concept that development consists of inherited historical processes is the degree to which such a plan can accomodate to environments that are not fully predictable. Since the natural environment contains so many changing features involving climate, food supply, predators, etc., flexibility or adaptability itself becomes of enormous selective advantage rather than too high a degree of specialization in adult forms. But if early environments can be controlled, predictable and reliably inherited, then specializations uniquely suited to these environments will be selected. Mammals have employed both these strategies by utilizing highly predictable early environments that are directly inherited (they involve first the mother's uterus and then the micro-environment of the parent's body) to promote the development of a relatively flexible and adaptive juvenile and adult with extraordinary learning capacities relative to other animals. The uterus, the breast and the social group are the three major inherited environments of the developmental plan which the process of evolution has given to mammals. It is our sequential adaptations to each of these which have been selected, but the intrauterine environment is the most highly specified and thus has elicited the most specialized adaptations.

The position of the mammalian fetus within the mother's body and the direct communication afforded by placental transfer allow maternal systems to regulate fetal physiology by the transfer of biologically active substances of many kinds in addition to the vital blood gases, oxygen and carbon dioxide: nutrients, amino acids, monoamine transmitters, neuro-active peptides, some steroid hormones and antibodies, enzymes and vitamins (Page, Villee & Villee, 1981). Only the largest molecules (e.g., cholesterol, phospholipids) and plasma protein conjugated substances are excluded by the placental membrane. Most drugs and toxins pass easily to the fetus. Thus the mother exerts physiological control of the developing fetus over a wide network of blood-borne regulatory substances which are gradually becoming elucidated. The distinctive tissue and biochemical abnormalities found in newborns of diabetic and nutrient deprived mothers are well known examples of these multiple regulatory effects (Fanaroff & Martin, 1983).

Much less is known about maternal influences upon fetal behavior. We have recently learned that in the late intrauterine period, the mother's voice appears to influence the systems responsible for auditory recognition and preference so that her voice is uniquely effective in eliciting behavior from her newborn child (see Fifer & Moon, this volume). Stephen Reppert and his coworkers (see Reppert & Weaver, this volume) have shown that pregnant dams of rodent and primate species set the phase of the fetal circadian pacemaker for the daily rhythms of activity, sleep and other functions that will not develop until the postnatal period. Other maternal-fetal regulatory influences on later infant behavior have been described, most of them involving blood borne factors such as hormones, nutrients, components of the immune system and ingested chemicals, including drugs of abuse which are transferred to the fetus by the placental circulation. The periodic uterine contractions, the secretions of the fetal membranes, the body movements of the mother in space, and the sounds (and lights) of the mother's chosen environment are less well studied pathways over which maternal regulation of fetal processes may take place (Hofer, 1981).

One of the possible adaptive functions of these pathways for direct maternal regulation is to preadapt the fetus to non-predictable features of the postnatal environment. Certain features of the mother's experience can be transferred to the fetus by processes other than learning. The fetal pacemaker example (above) illustrates this point: changes in phase and duration of environmental demands or light schedules can be conveyed to the fetus, preadapting it to seasonal aspects of the postnatal environment. The transgenerational effects of protein-calorie malnutrition is another example. Animal and human evidence demonstrates that the offspring of mothers which were malnourished in the fetal and infantile period have reduced brain and body size, and altered metabolism and activity levels. This occurs even if their mothers were fed normally in adulthood and throughout pregnancy. These effects are discernible for several generations after a single period of malnutrition in the first generation and are thought to involve placental, uterine and hormonal mechanisms (for recent review see Galler, 1988). The survival value of this form of transgenerational effect is clear, since the offspring are physiologically suited to the low levels of available food supply that are predicted by the previous generation's experience. (I should emphasize that although these are examples of the inheritance of acquired characteristics, they do not appear to involve genetic mechanisms.)

It is interesting to note that maternal regulation of infant physiological processes is not limited to the intrauterine period. Levels of a number of behavioral and physiological functions of infant rats are regulated by various different aspects of the mother-infant interaction during the postnatal period in which mother and infant remain in close proximity (Hofer, 1987). These influences are present even at an age when the infant is capable of survival on its own and only subside with dissolution of the close attachment between mother and offspring in the juvenile period. So here again, there is a continuity in the developmental processes between the intrauterine and the postnatal periods.

A possible adaptive function of these multiple maternal regulatory systems, in addition to the intergenerational transfer of information, is that their presence may have permitted the evolution of a number of fetal specializations that would be impossible in egg laying species. For if the embryo need not carry out all its own regulatory processes from within, this should make available control circuitry and the associated energy sources for application to other developmental processes such as the formation of neural structures capable of carrying out higher cognitive processes in postnatal life. I know of no clear evidence that control circuitry is a limited resource for the embryo, but it seems possible that in this way the evolution of extensive maternal regulation of the fetus by mammals may have played a role in the evolution of the advanced cognitive capabilities of the human brain. Certainly the rate and consistency with which energy and nutrients can be supplied during early development are facilitated by viviparity and contribute to the capacity for the elaboration of complex tissues such as the brain.

The intrauterine setting thus provides a highly predictable environment, isolated from the vicissitudes of the parent's ecological niche and replete with sources for regulation of the fetus's vital functions. These characteristics provide the inherited environment within which specific ontogenetic adaptations have evolved that give the behavior of the fetus its special character. *In utero*, the neural functions underlying sensory processes and behavior need not serve the requirements of exploiting and adapting to a complex and rapidly changing environment. They are instead available for another purpose.

EARLY NEURAL FUNCTION

Given the perspective I have outlined above, it becomes possible to approach the question of the function of prenatal behavior in a new light. The major developmental task of the fetal period is the formation of organized cellular systems and their integration into a functioning organism. The protection, the isolation from environmental perturbations and the steady supply of nutrient and of multiple regulatory controls that are afforded by the intrauterine environment, together support the vast organizational enterprise of building a highly complex nervous system, as described in the previous sections. But it has not yet been sufficiently appreciated that early neural function makes a significant contribution to that organizational enterprise. The idea that function can be in part responsible for structure turns on its head the usual sequence that we have come to accept. And yet, as I will describe below, that is what recent evidence from studies of neural development and prenatal behavior are forcing us to realize.

In the special period of ontogeny that takes place in utero, one of the major adaptive values of early neural function and behavior seems to be its usefulness in modifying the size, shape, composition and internal organization of developing neural and muscular organs at the tissue, cell and molecular levels. The developmental processes that are responsible for the creation of the neuromuscular system do not first build the structure and later set it in motion shortly before birth. Rather, the neural elements start to function very early and that activity plays numerous critical roles in determining the specific nature of the structures that subsequently develop, even in organs outside of the nervous system itself. The extent of such effects is radically reduced in the postnatal period so that, in this way, the behavior of the fetus can be considered as an ontogenetic adaptation.

Prenatal behavior is one of the sculptors of the organism and plays an essential role in accomplishing the task required of this stage in ontogeny by evolution: the building of an organism. A review of the many ways in which early neuronal function determines its structural design is beyond the scope of this article (for review, see Purves & Lichtman, 1985). But certain general principles and a few examples will be helpful in order to give some substance to this aspect of the role of prenatal behavior. The formation of organized structures of any sort from an undifferentiated early embryo depends on cell-cell communication so that each migrating cell will find its proper position and (partly as a result of its position) differentiate into its characteristic specialized form. Neurones proliferate, migrate and grow using chemical cues as do cells of other organ systems. But neurones also develop axonal and dendritic outgrowths so that networks of extremely long, branched cells are formed that are capable of communicating over long distances by electrochemically propagated nerve impulses.

Evidence of neural activation of embryonic muscle target cells can be recorded very early, even before definitive synapses are evident in electron microscopical sections (Dennis, Ziskind-Conhaim & Harris, 1981), and at a time when the axon terminal still has the appearance of the 'growth cone' which characterizes the leading point of cellular outgrowth. In the developing limb bud of a chick, for example, muscles begin to show spontaneous electrophysiological responses even before the primordial muscle mass has cleaved to form discrete muscles (Landmesser & Morris, 1975). Thus, neural activity starts when the first signs of structural differentiation begin to appear in the neuromuscular system, and thus is present as a potential influence on structure from the very beginning.

The other major function of neurones which starts very early is the axonal transport of so-called "trophic factors." Together with neural activity, these are the two major means by which neurones affect the formation of the specialized structures by which all elements of the nervous system communicate (synapses) and through which further effects on muscles and sense organs are subsequently exerted. The neurotransmitters released by neural activity also can act as trophic factors, thus linking the two processes. Trophic factors also are transported from target tissues (e.g. muscles) to neural cell bodies by axonal transport and act to stabilize connections and even to spare regional groups of neurones from the waves of cell death which occur periodically in certain regions of the developing nervous system.

Looking further along the neural output pathways, when a fetus's developing muscle is deprived of its neurally stimulated activity, a series of structural changes ensue. The most obvious of these is atrophy, a decrease in the diameter of each muscle fiber through loss of its major protein structure consisting of actin and myosin. The muscle fiber membrane also shows a number of biochemical and physiological changes: for example, the spreading out of acetylcholine receptors from the synapse over the whole surface of the muscle, and the appearance of periodic twitches called fibrillation. These changes occur in developing muscle deprived selectively of nerve activity by agents that prevent only neural impulses but not axonal transport of trophic substances (Drachman, 1968). The early start and long duration of intermittent muscle contraction during the prenatal period also plays a role in determining later specialized differentiation of individual muscle fiber types: either "slow twitch" or "fast twitch" functional classes, reflecting the differing biochemical characteristics of each type of muscle. During naturally occurring behaviors, fast twitch muscles are most efficient at sudden short-term movements while slow twitch muscles are most effective in situations where more prolonged contractions are required. Recent experiments employing long-term experimental manipulation of the frequency of nerve impulse activity to muscles have demonstrated that fast or slow twitch properties of muscles are produced by the frequency pattern of impulses delivered by the neurons innervating them (Salmons & Sreter, 1976).

Beyond effects of fetal neural activity on characteristics of the muscles, the first appearance of the joint spaces and the fine sculpting of the articular surfaces of the joints are a direct result of the limb movements that constitute fetal behavior. In chronically paralyzed chicks, Drachman and co-workers (1966) found that the cellular processes resulting in the orientation of cells and the thinning of cell layers on both sides of the developing joint and the loosening of tissue within the joints took place normally despite the prolonged lack of muscle activity. Tiny discontinuous spaces became visible within this loosening matrix, but instead of extending and fusing to form joint cavities, in paralyzed chicks this region filled with vascular connective tissue and finally the bones on either side became united by fibrous or cartilaginous bands which literally froze the limb joints in the fetal position. The articular surfaces of the bones were flattened and distorted so that only one limb position was possible. Some sesamoid bones (e.g., kneecap) remained fixed to the lower limb a long distance from the joints at which they are normally found. Finally, the intra-articular ligaments of the knee and ankle also failed to develop in the paralyzed limbs. Muscle characteristics of severe atrophy, as described above, completed the picture. These changes were found to occur equally readily after several different methods of inducing paralysis, showing that they were not merely side effects of any one method used. As a result of not being active in the egg, these chicks were structurally incapable of effective behavior after hatching. Similar experimental results have been reported in a mammal, the rat, by Moessinger (reviewed in this volume), and clinical evidence suggests that similar deficits may occur in humans (Hall, 1986).

Does early function also play a role in sensory or afferent systems? The development of specialized sensory structures such as the taste buds and the olfactory epithelium is dependent on their being innervated by sensory nerves; motor nerve innervation generally cannot substitute. The precise mechanisms underlying these effects have not been extensively studied, but since sensory organs are not activated by synapses, the influence of early neural connection is likely to be determined by chemical (trophic) factors, possibly delivered by the early developing neural function of axoplasmic transport. However, the evidence for the effects of neural activity in organizing and maintaining *central* sensory processing systems in the brain is extensive and compelling (Frank, 1987). Synaptic arrangements of subcortical and cortical cells, segregated functional units called "bands", "columns" or "barrels" depending on their shapes, begin to take place during the prenatal period. These specialized network structures allow information from individual sensory receptors to be processed by a particular set of neurons. Of course, most of the environmentally-tuned aspects of this organization take place postnatally. But there is considerable evidence of prenatal effects as well. Even in a system like the visual that receives little or no stimulation during the prenatal period, removal of the eye prenatally causes the cortical columns normally activated by that eye to shrink, whereas the columns from the opposite eye persist (Rakic, 1981).

Various forms of competition between neurons for trophic support also drive the diverse rearrangements of developing synapses that occur within central and peripheral neural structures. Here, not only the amount of activity but its timing may be crucial. For example, Hubel and Wiesel obtained evidence more than 20 years ago (1965) that asynchronous activity from the two eyes enhances competition between axons projecting to a single cortical neuron, while synchronous activity reduces or nullifies it, allowing the selective persistence of axon terminals that are repeatedly involved in synchronous (binocular) activation. This idea that specific synaptic patterns underlying the circuitry of the mature brain are determined by competition based on the timing of neural activity has had widespread usefulness in studies of developing autonomic ganglion cells and skeletal muscle as well as of sensory cortex (Purves & Lichtman, 1985, pp. 290–295).

In summary, for simple animals, the fates of individual cells during development tend to be rigidly controlled, whereas in vertebrates, with more complex brains, and mammals in particular, the ultimate nature and interconnections of neuromuscular and sensory cells are more flexible. Cell position and local chemical signals strongly influence this process, but early neural impulse conduction, together with neuronal transport of trophic substances, act in a variety of ways to shape and organize the developing tissues of the brain, the muscles, the sensory end organs, and even the joints of the limbs. These sculpting actions of early neural function are made possible by the special characteristics of the intrauterine environment. Given this perspective, we no longer have to explain *every* early behavior or sensory capability as having an anticipatory or preparatory function, and regressions of structure such as early cell death, and regressions of function, such as 'primitive' reflexes, can be understood as transient ontogenetic adaptations.

BEHAVIORAL STATE ORGANIZATION

As described above, the behavior of the fetus is not to be understood primarily in relation to its environment, as is the case with postnatal behavior, but in relation to its own development, as a component of the developmental process. This allows us to understand the relative absence of the goal-directed 'purposeful' character that we are accustomed to seeing in mammalian behavior. There is, however, a temporal patterning in neural activity from the outset in early fetal life, a cycling between activity and rest that provides continuity between prenatal and postnatal behavior. Beginning at the level of the individual neuron, activity levels fluctuate periodically as the outcome of biochemical processes within each cell and its local environment. Assemblages of interconnected neurons then begin to function as units with their own characteristics patterns of waxing and waning levels of activity resulting from inhibitory and excitatory feedback connections. Finally these local circuits come under the control of more centrally located groups of cells, which impose their own periodic patterns. This gathering together of units from within the broad matrix of early diffuse activity tends to organize the nervous system into a hierarchial structure of temporal patterning. As central excitatory and inhibitory systems gradually gain control over musculoskeletal, autonomic and neuroendocrine activity, functional patterns involving several systems become defined and the first behavioral state of the embryo can be identified.

In the human, two major trends characterize the development of state organization during gestation from 24 weeks to full term at 40 weeks: (a) the appearance and increased duration of quiescent periods, and (b) the increasingly close association of specific patterns of body movements with specific patterns of function in other systems as indicated by respiration, eye movements, electroencephalogram (EEG), heart rate, and electromyogram (EMG). Most of this data was first recorded in prematurely born infants (Dreyfus-Brisac, 1968; Parmalee & Stern, 1972), but recent ultrasound and heart rate recordings of fetuses in utero (Nijhuis, Martin & Prechtl, 1984) support the earlier findings. By 28–30 weeks, repetitive bursts of eye movements appear for the first time. These occur most often in association with the jerky body movements, irregular respiration, and very low EMG level that have been characteristic of the fetus for several weeks. Although the EEG is still primitive, most of the criteria for rapid eye movement or REM sleep are now present. The periods of motor quiescence are still not at all typical of later quiet or slow-wave sleep because respiration remains irregular, EMG is low, and slow waves can not yet be seen in the EEG. The association of patterned functioning that will become slow wave sleep develops between 32 and 40 weeks by a gradual prolongation of the periods during which no eye movements and few body movements occur. Behaviors consistent with the awake state begin to appear with the opening of the eyes at about 30 weeks gestation and become more clear cut with the association of sustained muscle tone and characteristic heart rate variability at about 36 weeks.

These states thus serve as integrating mechanisms for coordinating the disparate physiological and behavioral systems of the early fetus into functionally useful combinations. It is currently thought that wakefulness and the two sleep states each have different functions in the overall economy of the organism, predisposing for example to sustained activity, rest or memory consolidation (Webb, 1983). This allows different overall modes of functioning to be carried out by the same organism, a capacity which may be useful to the fetus and which it must develop in anticipation of the postnatal world. For example, the basic sleep-wake cycle allows both the fetus and the older infant to alternate between specialized programs for the discharge and for the reaccumulation of energy stores. Circadian state rhythms become temporally coordinated with environmental demands in the postnatal world by processes beginning prenatally (see Reppert & Weaver, this volume). In addition, the periodic cycling of these states provides the fetus with a changing set of internal conditions, despite the prevailing constancy of the intrauterine environment. These repeated transitions become progressively more sharply defined, so that by 38—40 weeks of gestation nearly all the parameters of each state are changing simultaneously. Though speculative, it seems likely that the long history of prenatal state shifts is utilized somehow in the developmental plan to prepare integrative central systems for adapting rapidly and precisely to sudden changes in the postnatal environment.

The first state that the human fetus develops is a state which most closely resembles REM sleep, and it spends 70—80% of its time in this state at 32 weeks of gestation. At term, this proportion declines to 50% and by 6 months postnatal age to 30%. Roffwarg and co-workers (1966), who were the earliest investigators to describe REM sleep in newborn infants, asked why so much of the early development of mammals is spent in the REM state and they proposed a hypothesis which continues to intrigue developmentalists. They noted that the REM state, from its first manifestations in the fetal period, is characterized by diffuse activating volleys from the brain stem to higher cortical centers and by localized phasic bursts of activation notably of eye muscles, but also of ear muscles, heart rate, blood pressure and other organs. But this intense activation is not expressed in overt behavior, except for localized minor muscle twitches, because of the superimposition of a generalized powerful inhibition of muscle tone. This intense internal activation, in an otherwise passive organism, seemed to suggest that it might represent a solution to a paradoxical evolutionary 'requirement' for activation without overt activity. Roffwarg postulated that such activation might be necessary in some way for the support of large masses of neural tissue that could not be directly involved in motor and sensory tasks during a relatively stable and protected early development. He called on embryologists to "give consideration to the possibility that REM sleep plays a role in stimulating structural maturation and maintenance within the central nervous system" (Roffwarg et al, 1966, p. 617).

A large body of neuroembryologic evidence has accumulated since Roffwarg's article, as reviewed in the previous section, and has provided us with a number of examples of cellular processes by which REM activation could exert the facilitating effects he postulated. Recently, two experimental studies have specifically implicated REM activation in neural development of the visual system. Davenne and Adrien (1985) made electrolytic lesions that interrupted the pathways for REM activation of the lateral geniculate nucleus (LGN) within the visual pathway of kittens, and found that the structural and physiological maturation of cells in that nucleus were impaired. Most recently Oksenberg and co-workers in Roffwarg's lab (1987) selectively deprived kittens of REM sleep by a non-invasive behavioral awakening procedure and found morphological effects in the LGN which were similar to those seen during deprivation of environmental light stimulation by eyelid occlusion.

It appears likely that the organization of neural activity into states in the last trimester of pregnancy in the human is not only evidence of neural maturation but also acts in a number of ways to facilitate neural development. REM sleep in the fetus may represent an example, at the level of integrative physiology, of the ontogenetic adaptation whereby early neuronal function acts as a vital ingredient in the developmental plan of the nervous system. Presumably, as the infant grows older, its interaction with the environment increasingly take the place of this state-specific internal stimulation. From its peak in the late fetal period, REM sleep proportion declines rapidly during the first postnatal year, possibly representing the decline of its role in neural development.

CONCLUDING SUMMARY

The realization that development is not simply a progressive unfolding, but instead embodies a number of processes that have evolved primarily in relation to the special environments and capabilities of the young organism, gives us a new way to approach questions about the nature and function of fetal behavior. Evolutionary processes have selected those characteristics of very young organisms that tend to solve two related but different needs: for the progressive building of an organism and for successful adaptation to immediate ecological requirements.

The intrauterine environment not only provides protection and constant supportive conditions, but also contributes specific regulators of the fetus's vital functions. The early behavior and 'precocious' latent perceptual and learning abilities of the fetus are not only preparatory in nature, but reflect another process. Newly differentiated neurons are capable of initiating impulse activity and axonal transport of trophic substances necessary for growth and maturation. Early in prenatal development, these neural functions play a role in the selective preservation and elimination of basic units such as neurons, synapses and muscle proteins. Later, the role of fetal neural activity is one of directing the arranging and rearranging of synaptic connections throughout the brain and of the structure of certain peripheral tissues such as muscles, joints and cartilage. Finally, the fetal REM state appears to supply a source for the required neural activation of cortical and subcortical brain areas that would not otherwise be stimulated within the relatively protected and stable environment of the intrauterine and early postnatal periods of life.

Acknowledgements

The author is supported by a Research Scientist Award from the National Institute of Mental Health.

References

Davenne, D., & Adrien, J. (1985) Electrophysiological maturation of the lateral geniculate neurons after lesion of the ponto-geniculo-occipital (PGO) pathways in the kitten. *Comptes Rendus de l'Academie des Sciences*, *300*, 59−64.

Dennis, M. J., Ziskind-Conhaim, L., & Harris, A. J. (1985). Development of neuromuscular junctions in rat embryos. *Developmental Biology*, *81*, 266−279.

Drachman, D. B., & Sokoloff, L. (1966). The role of movement in embryonic joint development. *Developmental Biology*, *14*, 401−420.

Drachman, D. B. (1968). The role of acetylcholine as a trophic neuromuscular transmitter. In G. E. W. Wolstenholme & M. O'Connor, (Eds.), *Ciba Foundation Symposium on Growth of the Nervous System*, (pp. 251−278). Boston: Little Brown.

Dreyfus-Brisac, C. (1968). Sleep ontogenesis in early human prematurity from 24−27 weeks of conceptual age. *Developmental Psychobiology*, *1*, 162−169.

Fanaroff, A. A., & Martin, R. J., (Eds.) (1983) Behrman's *Neonatal-Perinatal Medicine: Diseases of the Fetus and Infant*. 3rd Ed., St. Louis: C. V. Mosby.

Frank, E. (1987). The influence of neuronal activity on patterns of synaptic connections. *Trends in Neuroscience*, *10*, 188−189.

Galler, J. R. (1988). Nutrition and intergenerational effects. In *Understanding Mental Retardation: Research Accomplishments and New Frontiers*. Baltimore, MD: Paul H. Brookes.

Hall, J. G. (1986). Analysis of the Pena Shokeir phenotype. *American Journal of Medical Genetics*, *25*, 99−117.

Hall, W. G. (1975). Weaning and growth of artificially reared rats. *Science*, *190*, 1313−1315.

Hall, W. G., & Williams, C. L. (1983). Suckling isn't feeding or is it? A search for developmental continuities. *Advances in the Study of Behavior*, *13*, 218−254.

Hofer, M. A. (1981) *The Roots of Human Behavior: An Introduction to the Psychobiology of Early Development*. New York: W. H. Freeman.

Hofer, M. A. (1987). Shaping forces within early social relationships. In N. Krasnegor, E. Blass, M. Hofer & W. Smotherman, (Eds.), *Perinatal Development: A Psychobiological Perspective*, (pp. 251−274). Orlando: Academic Press.

Hubel, D. H., & Wiesel, T. N. (1965). Binocular interaction in striate cortex of kittens reared with artificial squint. *Journal of Neurophysiology*, *28*, 1041−1059.

Landmesser, L., & Morris, D. G. (1975). The development of functional innervation in the hind limb of the chick embryo. *Journal of Physiology* (*London*), *249*, 301−326.

Nijhuis, J. G., Martin, C. B., & Prechtl, H. F. R. (1984). Behavioral states of the human fetus. In H. F. R. Prechtl, (Ed.), *Continuity of Neural Functions From Prenatal to Postnatal Life*, (pp. 65−78). Philadelphia: Lippincott.

Oksenberg, A., Marks, G., Farber, J., Cobbey, K., Speciale, S., Mihailoff, G., & Roffwarg, H. (1987). REM sleep deprivation in kittens: Behavioral and pharmacological approaches. *Sleep Research*, *16*, 532.

Oppenheim, R. W. (1981). Ontogenetic adaptations and retrogressive processes in the development of the nervous system and behaviour: A neuroembryological perspective. In K. J. Connolly, & H. F. R. Prechtl, (Eds.), *Maturation and Development: Biological and Psychological Perspectives*, (pp. 73−109). Philadelphia: J. B. Lippincott Co.

Oyama, S. (1985). *The Ontogeny of Information: Developmental Systems and Evolution.* Cambridge: Cambridge Univ. Press.

Page, E. W., Villee, C. A., & Villee, D. B. (1981) *Human Reproduction: Essentials of Reproductive and Perinatal Medicine.* 3rd Ed. Philadelphia, PA: W. B. Saunders.

Parmalee, A. H., & Stern, E. (1972). Development of states in infants. In D. C. Clemente, D. P. Purpura & F. E. Mayer, (Eds.), *Sleep and the Maturing Nervous System*, (pp. 199−228). New York: Academic Press.

Preyer, W. (1885). *Physiologie des Embryo.* Leipzig.

Purves, D., & Lichtman, J. W. (1985). *Principles of Neural Development.* Sunderland, MA: Sinauer Assoc.

Raff, R. A., & Kaufman, T. C. (1983). *Embryos, Genes and Evolution.* New York: MacMillan.

Rakic, P. (1981). Development of visual centers in the primate brain depends on binocular competition before birth. *Science, 214,* 928−931.

Roffwarg, H., Muzio, J. N., & Dement, W. (1966). Ontogenetic development of the human sleep-dream cycle. *Science, 152,* 604−619.

Salmons, S., & Sreter, F. A. (1976). Significance of impulse activity in the transformation of skeletal muscle type. *Nature, 263,* 30−34.

Webb, W. (1983). Theories in modern sleep research. In A. Mayer, (Ed.), *Sleep Mechanisms and Functions in Humans and Animals*, (pp. 1−15). United Kingdom: Van Nostrand Reinhold.

Dimensions of Fetal Investigation

William P. Smotherman   and   Scott R. Robinson
Department of Psychology
State University of New York
Binghamton, New York

INTUITIVE VIEWS OF THE FETUS

The notion that the fetus can sense its environment and behave has received something of a bad press, or at least presents a sensational image to the public mind. Mention of the possibility of prenatal experience in polite conversation is likely to evoke one of two extreme reactions. Some people view prenatal life as mystically connected to the familiar postnatal world of children and adults. Popular books have appeared recently that have promulgated such views, arguing that mothers and fathers can communicate through ESP with the unborn child, that a child's IQ can be elevated by a parent's thinking about science or math from the moment of conception, that adult fears and psychological disorders can be treated by recognizing or recreating the prenatal traumas that produced them. Views such as these are part of a thriving body of popular pseudoscience that has no factual support.

Possibly as a reaction to extreme pseudoscientific views of prenatal life and possibly because fetal existence is fundamentally alien to our perceptions of the external world, a conservative viewpoint of prenatal life at the opposite extreme is often defended by scientists and medical professionals. This perspective depicts the fetus as a passive agent that grows in an unchanging world buffered from environmental stimuli. The fetus sleeps during most of its existence before birth, exhibits only sporadic, reflexive movements, and is influenced only as a receiving object in an environment regulated by the mother. Only at the time of birth is the fetus transformed into an active and interactive organism.

The conservative view of the fetus emphasizes the irrelevance of events during the prenatal period for understanding postnatal behavior. The varied contributions to this volume strongly attest to the poverty of the conservative perspective. Indeed, numerous points of continuity have now been identified between prenatal and postnatal behavior. Understanding the behavior of the fetus will require adoption of the conceptual

19

alternative to the conservative view of the fetus, namely, extension of an epigenetic perspective to the prenatal period. Further we believe that broadening epigenetic concepts to encompass events before birth will increase our understanding of behavioral development in general.

NEWBORN BEHAVIORAL COMPETENCE

Seen from a historical perspective, the conservative view of the fetus resembles earlier concepts of the infant during the first few months after birth. Early psychologists such as William James expressed the opinion that newborn infants are born into a "blooming, buzzing confusion" without an ability to adjust or respond. The newborn was seen as unable to sense, respond or learn. Apart from a handful of rudimentary reflexes, such as sucking and rooting, the newborn exists at the mercy of its environment. In the past 20 years the field of child development has experienced a conceptual revolution. The newborn is no longer viewed as inept. The reason that our view of the newborn has changed so dramatically is not that infants have changed, but that investigators have become more proficient at asking questions. Rather than evaluating the newborn in terms of adult perceptual and behavioral abilities, research programs have addressed the issue of neonatal behavior and cognition by adapting experimental procedures to environmental stimuli and motor patterns that are relevant to the infant. This research strategy has yielded important demonstrations in infants only a few days or hours old of visual fixation and discrimination (Aslin, 1985), speech recognition (Fifer and Moon, this volume), selective attention (Rohrbaugh, 1984), habituation and associative learning (Bornstein, 1985), orientation to adult faces and imitation of facial expression (Meltzoff & Moore, 1985), and recognition of mother (Balough & Porter, in press). Infants are now widely recognized as having a diverse behavioral repertoire and sophisticated intellectual abilities to perceive and interact with their environment.

In recognizing the behavioral competence of the newborn, however, an important question frequently has been overlooked: what is the developmental origin of the abilities of the newborn? Many of the discoveries of newborn competence have come from developmental psychologists. By reasons of training, they are prohibited from access to the fetus as a subject for direct experimental examination. Perhaps for this reason the fetus has been conveniently ignored. At the same time, physicians have access to tools that would enable fetal study, and have made use of these tools in a diagnostic context, but for practical professional reasons have traditionally not asked questions about the behavioral biology of the fetus. It is logically possible that neonatal abilities arise spontaneously at the moment of birth without prior expression or experience. But given the nature of developmental processes, it seems more likely that the behavioral competence of the newborn has unrecognized antecedents rooted in the prenatal period (Smotherman & Robinson, 1987a).

EMPIRICAL STUDY OF THE FETUS

The present is a paradoxical time for fetal research. Concern for the viability and healthy development of fetuses and infants is stimulating the desire of both the public and the professional community to learn more about prenatal development. At the same time, concern has fostered an appreciation of the fetus as a sensitive, fragile organism. Recent court cases, in which lawsuits have been brought on the behalf of fetuses against women that have abused drugs during pregnancy or against individuals or corporations that have endangered or compromised fetal viability dramatize this concern (Morris, 1986). The ethical considerations engendered by our changing awareness have restricted the methods that can be used to study the human fetus. A solution to this paradoxical impediment to fetal research has emerged with the development of noninvasive technological means of monitoring and imaging the fetus in utero.

Two important technologies have come to be routinely used in clinical applications in the past 10−15 years. External fetal monitoring, which involves little more than the placement of a sensory transducer around the abdomen of a pregnant women, enables the recording of fetal heart rate and detection of gross fetal body movements. More precise information about the kinds of movements exhibited by the fetus is provided by real-time ultrasonography, in which the echoes of high-frequency sound pulses are used to define contours and surfaces within the body and thereby produce a video image of the fetus as it moves in utero (see Birnholz, this volume). These two innovations have created a window on human fetal development that has replaced earlier approaches, such as examination of aborted fetuses (Humphrey, 1952).

Experimentation with human fetuses remains an emotionally charged issue. Moreover, recent quidelines for the study of human fetuses and ethical considerations in general have placed limitations on the direct study of human fetuses. Therefore, comparative study of nonhuman animals is imperative for understanding fetal behavior. Hofer (1981) eloquently reinforces this point and summarizes the logic for studying nonhuman animals:

"In working with a phylogenetically less advanced mammal, the strategy cannot be to seek a precise replica of the human situation. Rather, the plan is to describe a relatively simple model system whose workings can be understood through analytic experiments within a reasonable time frame. The general principles and some of the basic processes discovered at work in this simple system then become the basis for formulating new hypotheses, more specific, clearer, simpler, and hopefully the kind that can be tested in other species, including the human (pp. 245–246)."

Studies of the behavioral biology of the rat fetus take advantage of such an animal model (Smotherman & Robinson, 1988). A pregnant rat is prepared by injecting a solution of lidocaine into the spinal cord, producing complete but reversible spinal anesthesia posterior to the site of injection. The prepared female is then placed in a temperature-controlled bath containing a buffered physiological saline solution and the uterus externalized into the benign fluid medium. Spontaneous fetal activity is directly observed through the transparent wall of the uterus. To permit more detailed analysis of motor behavior or fetal response to tactile or chemical stimulation, individual fetuses are observed while immersed within the bath, after removal from the uterus and surrounding membranes without interruption of umbilical circulation. Fetuses observed under these conditions remain healthy for an hour or longer, which permits the recording of detailed sequences of fetal behavior. When preserved on videotape, such behavioral records are available for playback and reanalysis by investigators working on diverse research problems (see Robinson & Smotherman, this volume). These methods have provided the technical tools with which to investigate the prenatal development of behavior in the rat fetus.

EPIGENETIC PERSPECTIVE OF PRENATAL BEHAVIOR

Technical innovations are undeniably important in providing access to the fetus (see also Moessinger, this volume). But equally important are the concepts that are brought to the study of prenatal behavioral development. Conceptual frameworks within which specific research questions are phrased have a powerful impact on the vitality and direction of progress within a particular field of research. A focus on a dichotomy between 'learned' and 'innate' behavioral patterns (Lehrman, 1970) and on the 'integration' or 'differentiation' of behavior from simple reflexes (Carmichael, 1970) has formerly dominated research on early development, to the detriment of the field as a whole. Chief among the concepts that have replaced these simple dichotomies is the perspective of behavioral epigenesis. An early proponent of the view that the ontogeny of behavior is not different in principle from that of morphology, Kuo (1967, p. 11) defined behavioral epigenesis as "a continuous developmental process from fertilization through birth to death, involving proliferation, diversification, and modification of behavior patterns both in space and in time, as a result of the continuous dynamic exchange of energy between the developing organism and its environment, endogenous and exogenous."

Several points can be identified as fundamental to an epigenetic perspective. (a) Information is exchanged in both directions between the organism and its environment. Not only does the environment influence the course of development of the organism, but behavior of the organism can alter features of the environment, thereby changing the nature of their interaction (see Hofer, this volume). It is important that the environment be construed in the broadest terms to include aspects external to the organism (such as physical stimuli) as well as features of the internal milieu (e.g., the biochemical state of the organism). (b) Development consists of a succession of phenotypes that are the product of a dynamic relationship between the organism and its environment, not a gradual elaboration of an architectural plan preconfigured in the genes. Throughout development the range of possible outcomes—behavioral potentials (Kuo, 1967)— is large relative to the diversity of actual phenotypes that are observed. Behavioral potentials narrow as development is channeled along 'preferred' pathways. A schematic map of the branching of these pathways is often depicted as a form of ontogenetic landscape (Figure 1). (c) Understanding behavioral development thus entails documenting the succession of phenotypes that arise between fertilization and death (description of normal development) and investigating the processes involved in transforming one phenotype into the next (as in the experimental production of behavioral 'neophenotypes'). Ideally, transforming processes may be expressed formally, either in mathematical terms (i.e., the ontogenetic mapping function discussed by Hailman, 1982) or as developmental rules (e.g., Fentress & McLeod, this volume). We believe that investigation of behavioral development will benefit when founded upon epigenetic principles such as these.

Perhaps it seems as though we are beating a dead horse to reiterate the need to adopt an epigenetic view of behavioral development (see also Oyama, 1985). But some existing explanations for why the fetus moves acknowledge epigenesis for morphological development but implicity reject epigenesis with regard to behavior. Two broad classes of explanation have been proposed to account for prenatal movement. One explanation maintains that the fetus moves for no purpose; prenatal behavior serves no adaptive function and is merely an epiphenomenon of the maturation

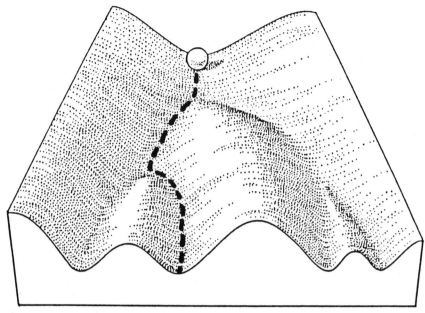

Figure 1. The "epigenetic landscape" as it applies to behavior. The ball signifies a pattern of behavior at an early point in development. Development progresses as the ball descends through the landscape. Factors that regulate/affect the pattern are represented by the locations, orientations and depths of the contours. (Adapted from C. H. Waddington. (1957). *The Strategy of the Genes*. London: Allen and Unwin.)

of nerves and muscles (see Provine, this volume). A necessary corollary to the perspective of fetal behavior as adaptively neutral is that birth is a critical event in ontogeny. The process of birth in some sense triggers the expression of remarkable perceptual and intellectual abilities in an adaptive context. This departure from the epigenetic perspective carries the implicit assumption that the behavioral abilities of the neonate are configurally preformed in emergent structure. In the alternative approach, behavioral development conforms to the same epigenetic processes that govern morphological development (Smotherman & Robinson, 1988). Ignoring the existence of prenatal behavior requires suspension of an epigenetic perspective of development, at least as it applies to behavior, for the entire period of ontogeny before birth.

THE ECOLOGY OF FETAL BEHAVIOR

Recent study of the behavioral biology of the fetus has provided a clear example of the dynamic exchange of information between the developing organism and its changing environment. The amniotic fluid that bathes the fetus is a principal component of the intrauterine environment throughout gestation. Shortly after the amniotic and chorionic membranes differentiate, they begin to produce the amniotic fluid that fills the cavity surrounding the embryo. The resulting environment physically buffers the developing embryo from mechanical stimuli (e.g., touch, sound) originating outside the mother and provides a medium in which the first movements of the fetus (which appear during weeks 7–8 of gestation in humans) can occur with little restriction. In contrast to this early period of development, in which the composition and amount of amniotic fluid are regulated by processes external to the fetus, older fetuses (during the second half of gestation) assume a more active role in the regulation of amniotic fluid volume, viscosity, and composition. Fetal behavior, which includes ingestion of fluid and micturition into the amniotic sac, is an important aspect of this regulation. Through its effects on amniotic fluid, the fetus comes to participate in the dynamics of its intrauterine environment.

Coincident with the involvement of the fetus in regulating amniotic fluid is a growing influence of the intrauterine environment on the expression of fetal behavior. As the volume of amniotic fluid diminishes relative to fetal body size, increasing physical restraint within the uterus begins to interfere with fetal movement. Amniotic fluid also changes in composition and specific chemical constituents exert an influence on the behavior of pups and neonates around the time of birth (Pedersen & Blass, 1982; Hepper, 1987). It is within the physically restricted environment of the uterus that the fetus begins to express behavioral organization and diversity (see chapters by Robertson, Reppert & Weaver, Robinson & Smotherman, this volume) and to exhibit particular patterns of behavior that are important to its well-being, such as turning to the normal vertex (head down) position prior to the onset of labor and delivery (Suzuki & Yamamuro, 1985). The interplay between the fetus and its fluid milieu thus changes over the course of gestation, illustrating the interdependence of emerging behavior and the environmental context in which it occurs (Smotherman & Robinson, 1988).

PROBLEMS IN THE IDENTIFICATION OF BEHAVIORAL ISOMORPHISM

Developmental researchers often take as their starting point a pattern of behavior that is evident in the adult of a species. The strategy is then adopted of seeking evidence of the adult pattern in immature individuals at progressively younger ages. At the most basic level, developmental milestones are catalogued. Identifying the earliest age at which a particular pattern of behavior is expressed is not necessarily a simple task. Two conflicting demands interact to shape the behavior of the developing organism. Much of development is preparatory; particular patterns of behavior emerge early to provide a period in which the pattern may be modified and perfected before it is needed in a functional context. At the same time that the immature organism is preparing for its future life, it must survive in its current environment. Structures and behavioral patterns emerge that are functional during only a limited period of ontogeny. Recognizing the distinction between preparatory behavior and ontogenetic adaptation is fundamental to understanding when behavioral patterns originate and explaining how they achieve their final form (Oppenheim, 1984).

There are pragmatic difficulties in determining whether similar patterns of behavior expressed early in development and later in adulthood are in fact isomorphic. This is a problem in identifying behavioral homology (Ghiselin, 1976). In comparative and evolutionary research, many forms of homology are recognized. In the most basic usage, two structures that are similar in different species are considered homologous if their similarity is a function of their common evolutionary heritage (i.e., the common ancestor also possessed the structure). Serial homology is the repeated expression of similar structures within an organism, such as vertebrae in the spinal column. Behavior poses special problems for comparison, as successive performances of behavioral patterns may differ; identifiable, repeatable action patterns in an individual have been referred to as iterative homology. But as behavior changes during development, similar actions can diverge and dissimilar actions come to resemble one another. In this way, the study of behavioral continuity during development, like the tracing of phylogenetic trees, is the principal method by which ontogenetic homologies can be recognized. Behavioral continuity, and thus the isomorphism or homology of similar patterns of behavior, is simplest to document when two instances of a behavioral pattern occur in close temporal proximity. But homology becomes increasingly difficult to document as the temporal separation of behavioral events increases. The degree of difference between an immature organism and the adult can be visualized as ontogenetic distance. It is most difficult to document behavioral homology when ontogenetic distance is greatest, and the greatest ontogenetic distance lies between the fetus and the adult.

There is an intellectual pitfall in adopting the view that a continuous developmental trace (i.e., expression at all ages) is needed to identify homology at large ontogenetic distances. Some patterns of behavior are indeed expressed continuously from their first appearance through adulthood. Other patterns, however, are exhibited at an early point during ontogeny, paradoxically disappear for a period of time, and subsequently reappear. At the same time, similarity of superficial form or function also is insufficient to identify developmental homology. Just as homologous structures in distantly related species may exhibit remarkably different forms, early patterns of behavior may appear quite different from their mature expression in adults. Conversely, patterns of behavior that are separated by a large ontogenetic distance may be accidentally similar and not continuous, the early pattern changing during development to give rise to an another pattern of adult behavior or disappearing completely, without issue. These patterns of ontogenetic change are well recognized in morphological development and should be considered logically equivalent alternatives in the study of behavioral development. Because early and mature patterns of behavior may be connected by different ontogenetic paths, developmental researchers must consider alternatives to the conventional conception of a continuous developmental trace between patterns of behavior that are outwardly similar. In the remainder of this essay, we will outline two examples of how alternative developmental patterns have been identified in behavioral research.

DEVELOPMENT OF BIPEDAL WALKING IN HUMANS

It has long been known that for the first few weeks after birth, human infants will exhibit a stepping "reflex" when supported in an upright posture with feet in contact with a substrate. Stepping by the newborn is remarkably similar to walking, but disappears about 6–8 weeks after birth. But the superficial similarity of neonatal stepping to walking is not sufficient to demonstrate developmental continuity. It has been argued, for example, that neonatal stepping is simply the expression of a pattern of behavior that was functional during the late prenatal period (perhaps to facilitate attainment of the vertex position by the fetus) and was incidentally retained into early postnatal life. By this view, neonatal stepping is an ontogenetic adaptation that coincidentally resembles walking but is not continuous with any pattern of adult behavior. During the interval between the disappearance of neonatal stepping and the beginning of the familiar progression from crawling to standing to walking in childhood, infants in a prone posture exhibit an assortment of (seemingly) non-directed leg movements. Thelen and Fisher (1982) have convincingly shown that these leg movements are not random, but exhibit organization in temporal and spatial dimensions. Although kicking by prone infants seems unrelated to vertically oriented walking motions, frame-by-frame analysis of fine motor organization, simultaneous recording of EMG from leg musculature, and recording of motivational context (states of arousal) reflect an underlying continuity of neonatal stepping, spontaneous leg movements by infants and later walking. Thus it is not the continuous expression of outwardly similar motor patterns at all intervening ages that links neonatal stepping with walking. Rather, it is the discovery of a superficially dissimilar pattern of behavior—organized spontaneous leg movements—that permitted the bridging of a period of apparent discontinuity to logically identify the underlying ontogenetic homology of neonatal stepping and bipedal walking.

DEVELOPMENT OF FACIAL WIPING IN RATS

In spite of the convincing demonstration of continuity between stepping and walking, animal models can provide the experimenter with ways to interact with the prenatal and postnatal environments that are not possible in the non-manipulative study of human fetuses and neonates. The fruitfulness of the experimental approach with non-human animal subjects is illustrated by recent progress in our understanding of the ontogeny of spontaneous and stimulus-evoked behavior in rat fetuses. Using techniques for direct observation following fetal stimulation (described above), we have found that the intraoral infusion of novel chemical solutions, such as lemon extract, consistently elicits a sudden increase in fetal activity on days 19−21 of gestation. As one aspect of the overall increase in motor activity, fetuses perform a rapid series of coordinated foreleg movements which contact the side of the head in a rostral direction (Figure 2). This facial wiping is nearly always elicited by lemon infusions on days 20 and 21 (Figure 3 top), but rarely occurs on day 19 of gestation (Smotherman & Robinson, 1987b). Fetal facial wiping is remarkably similar to postnatal grooming patterns that are exhibited during aversion sequences (Grill & Berridge, 1985), which suggests continuity between these patterns of prenatal and postnatal behavior.

The evident prenatal expression of a species-typical action pattern is more remarkable in view of earlier reports that rat pups do not develop facial wiping until the second week of postnatal life (Johanson & Shapiro, 1986). In independent replications, we have confirmed that pups are less likely than fetuses to perform wiping behavior in response to lemon infusion. Pups were tested within one hour of delivery by Caesarean section or one day after birth in an incubator regulated at typical nest temperature. One-day-old pups almost never performed facial wiping in response to lemon infusion. Newborn pups exhibited wiping more fre-

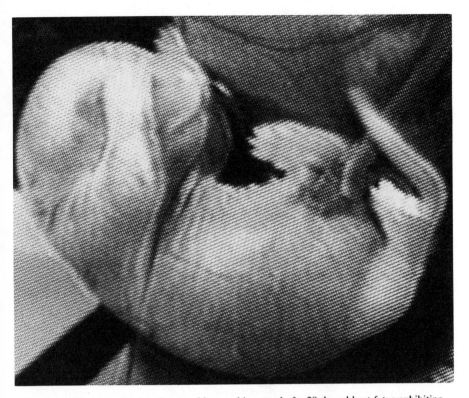

Figure 2. Photograph taken from a videographic record of a 20-day-old rat fetus exhibiting facial wiping in response to a 20 μl intraoral infusion of lemon.

quently than older pups, but less frequently than fetuses. Pups that did exhibit wiping in such a terrestrial environment did so only when in a lateral or supine posture. The diminished likelihood for older pups to wipe therefore may be a consequence of their greater ability to maintain a prone body posture. These observations fit well with the report by Golani and Fentress (1985) that one-day-old mouse pups will perform facial grooming movements if externally supported in an upright posture.

Manipulation of the conditions under which fetuses and neonatal rats are tested has provided further evidence that prenatal and postnatal facial wiping are continuous and has gone far toward explaining why young rat pups ordinarily do not exhibit this pattern of behavior. In the first of a series of experiments, some physical aspects of the prenatal environment were simulated by immersing neonatal rat pups below the neck in a warm water bath at the time of testing (see also Bekoff this volume; Bekoff & Kauer, 1984). Both on the day of birth and one day later, pups suspended in a fluid medium exhibited vigorous facial wiping in response to lemon

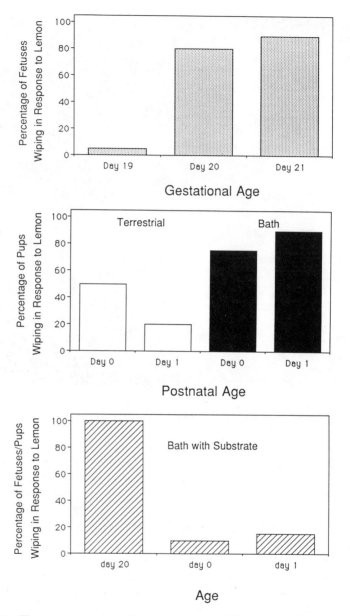

Figure 3. The percentage of rat fetuses or pups exhibiting facial wiping in response to lemon infusions. (Top) Wiping response of fetuses at three ages to infusion of lemon. (Middle) Wiping response of pups tested in a terrestrial environment or immersed in a warm saline bath. (Bottom) Wiping response of fetuses and pups tested in the bath on a submerged substrate.

infusion (Figure 3 Middle). This finding indicates that certain features of the postnatal environment normally constrain or inhibit the expression of facial wiping.

To investigate further which aspects of the environment are effective in reducing the expression of facial wiping, another group of pups were tested while immersed in the water bath. These pups were positioned with paws and ventral surface in contact with a submerged substrate prior to infusion. When tested under these conditions, both newborns and one-day-old rat pups responded to lemon infusions with increased activity, but exhibited facial wiping only rarely. Physical contact with a hard substrate, even in a buoyant aqueous medium, is sufficient to reduce the expression of postnatal facial wiping. The behavior of pups on a substrate thus provides further evidence for the environmental constraint of this species-typical action pattern.

The occurrence of wiping by newborn pups and its disappearance within 24 hours may be due to a gradual process of adaptation to features present in the terrestrial environment. As a beginning approach toward evaluating this idea, day 20 fetuses, which lack any experience with a terrestrial environment, were tested after placement on a submerged substrate (with intact placental attachment). The response of day 20 fetuses to lemon infusion while on a substrate was indistinguishable from that of fetuses tested off the substrate; all exhibited facial wiping during an overall increase in activity (Figure 3; bottom). An influence of the substrate is apparent 24 hours later, however, when only half of the fetuses tested on a submerged substrate exhibited a wiping response to lemon infusion. The results of testing fetuses on a substrate are consistent with the possibility of age-specific responsiveness to substrate cues, but also suggest that increased exposure of fetuses to features of the intrauterine environment that mimic the terrestrial environment promotes the development of substrate-induced inhibition of facial wiping (Smotherman & Robinson, in press). Collectively, these findings indicate that the facial wiping originally described for rat pups during the second week of life has prenatal origins. The apparent discontinuity between prenatal and postnatal wiping is a consequence of the neonatal rat's motor immaturity in the context of a gravitational environment (rat pups cannot maintain a posture in which the forelegs are free for facial wiping).

These findings, which seem surprising upon first appraisal, are consistent with current views of behavioral continuity and illustrate different patterns of behavioral homology as outlined above. In the course of normal development, facial wiping exhibits a pattern of presence (prenatal), absence (neonatal) and presence (older pups). The transient period of absence produced by environmental constraints obscures underlying continuity. In the development of bipedal locomotion in humans (Thelen & Fisher, 1982), as in the transition from aquatic to terrestrial locomotion in frogs (Stehouwer & Farel, 1985; see discussion in Thelen, this volume), early motor patterns are superficially dissimilar from mature patterns of locomotion, and sophisticated movement analysis or neurophysiological techniques are required to reveal underlying continuities. Conversely, neonatal suckling behavior and later ingestive behavior in rats appear similar and are expressed continuously during development. Yet close analysis of the development of feeding behavior has disclosed that suckling is more correctly viewed as an ontogenetic adaptation that is not a simple precursor of mature feeding behavior (Hall & Williams, 1983).

THIS VOLUME

We do not envision that the recent breakthroughs in recognizing behavioral sophistication in the fetus and the continuities between prenatal and postnatal life will result in a fundamental change of focus in developmental research. It is entirely appropriate that the principal emphasis of developmental investigation center on the postnatal period. After all, the majority of our lives fall after the moment of birth. But if this volume serves no other purpose, we hope it will highlight the simple ideas that (a) ontogeny is a cumulative process and (b) the organism begins the postnatal period with a rich experiential history. A more complete understanding of this history will provide an important missing piece toward completing the puzzle of behavioral development.

Acknowledgement

William P. Smotherman is supported by Grant HD 16102−06 and Research Career Development Award HD 00719−02 from the National Institute of Child Health and Human Development (NIH). The authors would like to thank Drs. Mary Gauvain and Peter Hepper for cogent comments on an earlier draft of this chapter.

References

Aslin, R. N. (1985). Oculomotor measures of visual development. In G. Gottlieb & N. A. Krasnegor (Eds.), *Measurement of audition and vision in the first year of postnatal life: a methodological overview* (pp. 391−417). Norwood, NJ: Ablex.

Balough, R. D. & Porter, R. H. (In press). Olfactory preferences resulting from mere exposure in human neonates. *Infant Behavior and Development*.

Bekoff, A. & Kauer, J. A. (1984). Neural control of hatching: fate of the pattern generator for the leg movements of hatching in post-hatching chicks. *Journal of Neuroscience, 11*, 2659–2666.

Bornstein, M. H. (1985). Habituation of attention as a measure of visual information processing in human infants: summary, systematization, and synthesis. In G. Gottlieb & N. A. Krasnegor (Eds.), *Measurement of audition and vision in the first year of postnatal life: a methodological overview* (pp. 253–300). Norwood, NJ: Ablex.

Carmichael, L. (1970). The onset and early development of behavior. In P. H. Mussen (Ed.), *Carmichael's manual of child psychology*, 3rd edition (pp. 447–563). New York: Wiley.

Ghiselin, M. T. (1976). The nomenclature of correspondence: a new look at "homology" and "analogy". In R. B. Masterton, W. Hodos & H. Jerison (Eds.), *Evolution, brain and behavior: persistent problems* (pp. 129–142). Hillsdale, NJ: Erlbaum.

Golani, I. & Fentress, J. C. (1985). Early ontogeny of face grooming in mice. *Developmental Psychobiology, 18*, 529–544.

Grill, H. J., & Berridge, K. C. (1985). Taste reactivity as a measure of the neural control of palatability. In J. M. Sprague & A. N. Epstein (Eds.), *Progress in psychobiology and physiological psychology*, vol. 11 (pp. 1–61). New York: Academic Press.

Hailman, J. P. (1982). Ontogeny: toward a general theoretical framework for ethology. In P. P. G. Bateson & P. H. Klopfer (Eds.), *Perspectives in ethology*, vol. 5, *ontogeny* (pp. 133–189). New York: Plenum.

Hall, W. G., & Williams, C. L. (1983). Suckling isn't feeding, or is it? A search for developmental continuities. In J. S. Rosenblatt, R. A. Hinde, C. Beer & M. C. Busnel (Eds.), *Advances in the study of behavior*, vol. 13 (pp. 219–254). New York: Academic Press.

Hepper, P. G. (1987). The amniotic fluid: an important priming role in kin recognition. *Animal Behaviour, 35*, 1343–1346.

Hofer, M. A. (1981). *The Roots of Human Behavior*. San Francisco: W. H. Freeman.

Humphrey, T. (1953). The relation of oxygen deprivation to fetal reflex arcs and the development of fetal behavior. *Journal of Psychology, 35*, 3–43.

Johanson, I. B., & Shapiro, E. G. (1986). Intake and behavioral responsiveness to taste stimuli in infant rats from 1 to 15 days of age. *Developmental Psychobiology, 19*, 593–606.

Kuo, Z. Y. (1967). *The Dynamics of Behavior Development*. New York: Random House.

Lehrman, D. S. (1970). Semantic and conceptual issues in the nature–nurture problem. In L. R. Aronson, E. Tobach, D. S. Lehrman & J. S. Rosenblatt (Eds.), *Development and evolution of behavior* (pp. 17–52). San Francisco: W. H. Freeman.

Meltzoff, A. N. & Moore, M. K. (1985). Cognitive foundations and social functions of imitation and intermodal representation in infancy. In J. Mehler & R. Fox (Eds.), *Neonate cognition: beyond the blooming, buzzing confusion* (pp. 139–156). Hillsdale, NJ: Erlbaum.

Morris, R. A. (1986). Legal implications for research in the developing organism. *Neurotoxicology, 7*, 3–18.

Oppenheim, R. W. (1984). Ontogenetic adaptations in neural and behavioural development: toward a more 'ecological' developmental psychobiology. In H. F. R. Prechtl (Ed.), *Continuity of neural functions from prenatal to postnatal life* (pp. 16–30). Oxford: Blackwell Scientific Publications.

Oyama, S. (1985). *The ontogeny of information: developmental systems and evolution*. Cambridge: Cambridge Univ. Press.

Pedersen, P. E. & Blass, E. M. (1982). Prenatal and postnatal determinants of the first suckling episode in albino rats. *Developmental Psychobiology, 15,* 349–355.

Rohrbaugh, J. W. (1984). The orienting reflex: performance and central nervous system manifestations. In R. Pavasuramam & D. R. Davies (Eds.), *Varieties of attention* (pp. 323–373). New York: Academic Press.

Smotherman, W. P. & Robinson, S. R. (1987a). Prenatal influences on development; behavior is not a trivial aspect of fetal life. *Journal of Developmental and Behavioral Pediatrics, 8,* 171–176.

Smotherman, W. P. & Robinson, S. R. (1987b). Prenatal expression of species-typical action patterns in the rat fetus. *Journal of Comparative Psychology, 101,* 190–196.

Smotherman, W. P. & Robinson, S. R. (1988). The uterus as environment: the ecology of fetal behavior. In E. M. Blass (Ed.), *Handbook of behavioral neurobiology,* vol. 9, *Developmental psychobiology and behavioral ecology* (pp. 149–196). New York: Plenum.

Smotherman, W. P. & Robinson, S. R. (in press). Cryptopsychobiology: the appearance, disappearance and reappearance of a species-typical action pattern during early development. *Behavioral Neuroscience.*

Stehouwer, D. J. & Farel, P. B. (1985). Development of locomotor mechanisms in the frog. *Journal of Neurophysiology, 53,* 1453–1466.

Suzuki, S. & Yamamuro, T. (1985). Fetal movement and fetal presentation. *Early Human Development, 11,* 255–263.

Thelen, E. & Fisher, D. M. (1982). Newborn stepping: an explanation for a 'disappearing' reflex. *Developmental Psychology, 18,* 760–775.

On The Uniqueness Of Embryos And The Difference It Makes

Robert R. Provine
Department of Psychology
University of Maryland Baltimore County
Baltimore, Maryland

A wide range of investigators from the neural and behavioral sciences are joining neuroembryologists in the study of prenatal development. Their motives are varied. Some are extending their developmental observations from the postnatal into the prenatal period. Others are interested in some aspect of embryogenesis. Yet others are using embryos to investigate non-developmental phenomena. These welcome recruits bring new techniques, ideas, and interests to the previously active, but underpopulated research area of prenatal studies. However, both newcomers and veteran embryologists are sometimes insensitive to some of the special properties of embryos and of the prenatal domain. Developmentalists have long understood that embryos are not simply smaller, unformed versions of the adult, but they have not always been alert to unique features and specializations of embryos, some of which are structural and functional adaptations to the prenatal environment (Oppenheim, 1981). The prenatal and postnatal forms of an organism, or even embryos at different developmental stages, are often so different in structure that were it not for an awareness of the thread of developmental continuity, they would seem to be members of different species. Less obvious but equally great differences between developmental stages exist at the physiological and behavioral levels.

The intent of the present essay is to encourage an appreciation of and search for unique properties of embryos.[1] This perspective is offered as a partial antidote for the tendency to impose preconceptions about prenatal development or adults on the embryo. To illustrate some of the special

---

[1] No distinction is made here between the often nebulous categories termed embryo and fetus. Unless otherwise noted, the term embryo refers to all prenatal developmental stages.

qualities of embryos, I describe three phenomena of neurobehavioral development that lack postnatal counterparts. None of these phenomena could have been predicted by extrapolating from the postnatal to the prenatal period. As noted above, the presence of such novel embryonic processes is not surprising. History has shown the embryo to be notoriously indifferent to the biases and expectations of philosophers, biologists, and psychologists who venture into the developmental arena.

SPONTANEOUS MOVEMENT AND ITS NEURAL CORRELATES

The history of the study of spontaneous embryonic movement is a fitting introduction to the problems that can arise when preconceptions about development take priority over observations in the study of behavior.

The scientific study of behavior development got off to a good start with the publication of Preyer's classic text on the *Specielle Physiologie des Embryo* (Preyer, 1885). One of the significant observations of Preyer was that the chick embryo moved several days before the first movements could be evoked. Thus, pre-reflexogenic movement was spontaneous. The ramifications of this important finding for behavior occurring after the onset of reflexes was neither fully appreciated nor pursued experimentally until the 1960's (Hamburger, 1963).

Another significant event in the neuroembryological study of behavior was Coghill's publication of *Anatomy and the Problem of Behavior* (1929) that summarized his long-term research of behavior development of the salamander *Ambystoma*. As suggested by his book's title, Coghill described behavioral events during development and attempted to correlate them with the appearance of neuroanatomical structures. On the basis of his observations of salamanders, he proposed a general theory of development that held behavior to be totally integrated at all ages and independent movements to emerge from a total pattern by a process that he called individuation. Coghill's proposal suffered the fate of many general accounts of behavior in that it extended an explanation that may have been appropriate for one species (*Ambystoma*) to other inappropriate ones. Later comparative analyses detected many exceptions to the individual model (Hamburger, 1963; Provine, 1986).

Another general model of behavior development was advocated by Windle on the basis of his observations of mammalian fetuses (Windle, 1940). He suggested that coordinated movements emerged through the integration of local reflex circuits. His emphasis of the reflex was in part due to the coincidence of the first reflexes and movements in mammalian fetuses. This finding was also consistent with the then prevalent view that behavior was the product of environmental stimulation. Because movement was considered to be evoked, ongoing behavior was either neglected or considered to be a response to unidentified stimuli. Subsequent analyses demonstrated that the reflex, the key element of Windle's system, and a construct dear to the radical environmentalists of the day, was not the basic unit of behavior in either the adult (Grillner, 1975) or the embryo (Provine, 1986).

The next major contribution to our understanding of spontaneous movement was made by Hamburger and colleagues in the 1960s, who combined behavioral observation with elegant microsurgical procedures to demonstrate the non-reflexogenic nature of embryonic motility of the chick.[2] In a classic study, Hamburger et al. (1966) extirpated several segments of the thoracic neural tube (immature spinal cord) to isolate the lumbosacral spinal cord from brain input. Simultaneously, a second operation removed the dorsal half of the neural tube caudal to the thoracic spinal gap and the associated neural crest areas (the precursor of the dorsal root sensory ganglia), eliminating sensory input to the residual, postgap cord. The legs innervated by the isolated, deafferented lumbosacral spinal cord segment performed high levels of characteristic motility during most of the embryonic period. Thus, the leg movement of these experimental embryos and presumably most behavior of normal, intact embryos, was both spontaneous and generated by neuronal circuitry within the spinal cord. These results were surprising to many developmentalists for two reasons: embryonic behavior was the result of spontaneous, not evoked activity; and the spinal cord, not the brain, was the origin of the activity.

A theme running through research on embryonic neurobehavioral development is that many locomotor systems mature independently of sensory input, practice, and other sources of environmental instruction. Also, as first noted by Preyer (1885), the phenomenon of motor precocity indicates that motor systems develop before, and, therefore, without influence of their inputs. There are numerous physiological (Bruce and Tatton, 1980; Stein et al., 1980) and anatomical (Foelix and Oppenheim, 1973) examples of the early development of efferent relative to afferent processes. The presence of these retrograde developmental sequences

---

[2] The historically prominent research by Harrison, Carmichael, and others on the effects of rearing amphibians in paralyzing anesthetics will not be pursued here because it does not deal directly with the present topic of spontaneous behavior. Readers interested in this research are referred to Haverkamp (1986) and Haverkamp and Oppenheim (1986) who provide new data and scholarly reviews that resolve several controversies indigenous to this area.

indicates that sensation, motivation, and learning are much less significant for embryos than for the organism after birth.

About 1970, neurophysiology was added to the more traditional behavioral and anatomical methods that were used to study problems of behavior development.[3] Electrical recordings from paralyzed (curarized) and motile chick embryos confirmed the role of the spinal cord in the production of spontaneous movement and revealed some novel phenomena of embryonic neurophysiology (Provine, 1972, 1973). Massive polyneuronal burst discharges were identified within the ventral cord region (Provine et al., 1970) shown by Hamburger et al. (1966) to produce motility in spinal deafferented embryos. The bursts were synchronized with embryonic movements in motile embryos and with motor nerve discharges in curarized preparations (Ripley and Provine, 1972). When a burst occurred, the embryo moved; embryonic movements never occurred in the absence of a simultaneous burst.

Aside from their obvious significance as neural correlates of embryonic motility, the spinal cord burst discharges are interesting in their own right. Spinal cord bursts usually begin with a high amplitude "initiating" discharge that is usually followed by a longer, lower amplitude, and more variable "afterdischarge". Before 7 days of embryonic age, bursts consist only of "initiating" discharges (Provine, 1972, 1973). The increase in burst duration and complexity between 6 and 7 days has been confirmed in recordings from the ventral root of the isolated spinal cord (O'Donovan and Landmesser, 1987). As noted by Landmesser and O'Donovan (1984), the initiating and afterdischarge pattern of burst discharge (which they refer to as synchronous and delayed discharges) may be unique to the embryo.

The electromyographic work of Bekoff (1976) and Landmesser and O'Donovan (1984) is useful in understanding how the spinal cord bursts translate into the contraction of specific muscles. Their electromyograms suggest that the initiating component of a burst usually triggers activity in all muscles. Differences between the activity of different muscles occur

---

[3] Embryologists are traditionally trained in anatomical methods. The science of anatomy benefited from this association. The study of embryology brought dynamism, a functional orientation, and experimental procedures to classical, descriptive anatomy. The traditional approach of experimental embryology was to observe the structural consequences of surgical isolation, transplantation and extirpation to discover the determinants of morphogenesis. The passing of the "golden age" of anatomically oriented experimental embryology roughly coincided with the ascendence of biochemistry and molecular biology.

primarily during the burst afterdischarge. In the spinal cord, the afterdischarge is also responsible for the differences between bursts observed simultaneously at different cord sites (Provine, 1971).

Concurrent recordings from two electrodes at different spinal cord sites indicate that a given burst occurs almost simultaneously along the rostrocaudal axis of the cord (Provine, 1971). The small but variable latencies between the onset of bursts at different regions suggest that bursts are initiated at varying cord loci and then propagated throughout the remainder of the cord. This inherent burstiness and transregional coupling of discharges is not typical of the postnatal spinal cord. The presence of such spontaneous spinal cord bursting and correlated muscular twitches after birth would produce behavioral chaos on which would be superimposed reflexes and voluntary movements.

The transregionally coupled burst discharges that are typical of the spinal cord, and perhaps other parts of the embryonic central nervous system, may provide a useful model of adult paroxysmal activity such as epilepsy. Indeed, some forms of epilepsy may even be produced by the postnatal remnant of normally bursty neuronal tissue, or by the return of previously quiescent tissue to the typically bursty, embryo-like state as a result of trauma or disease. A point in favor of this "embryonic" hypothesis of epilepsy is that it is based on a process normally present in embryos and does not require the poisons, trauma, or kindling necessary to produce postnatal seizures in other model systems. Recent reviews of experimental models of epilepsy (Porter, et al., 1984; Schwartzkroin and Wheal, 1983) do not consider this "embryonic" hypothesis.

ROLE OF SPONTANEOUS BEHAVIOR IN MUSCLE AND JOINT DEVELOPMENT

Studies of sensory enrichment and deprivation at postnatal stages indicate that environmental stimulation and "experience" can influence both behavior and its neural substrate (Hubel and Wiesel, 1970; Blakemore and Cooper, 1970). In contrast, the embryo seems largely indifferent to the contingencies of the sensory environment. The embryo is, however, highly attuned to another sort of environment. Textbooks of developmental biology are catalogues of the highly social relationships between the extended family of cells that is the embryo. The present section considers some novel consequences of embryonic movement that are behaviorally significant yet tend to fall into the cracks between disciplines and be overlooked. Embryonic movement has effects on muscle and joint development that are of a type seldom encountered by either embryologists concerned with the intercellular matrix or developmental psychologists concerned with the extraorganismic, sensory environment.

The function of ongoing motor activity can be evaluated by observing the consequences of paralyzing the embryo with neuromuscular blocking agents such as curare. As little as 24 to 48 hours of curare-induced paralysis produces permanent malformation of joints and atrophy of muscles in the chick embryo (Drachman and Sokoloff, 1966). (The effect of paralysis on motoneuron survival is explored in the next section of this paper). Therefore, early movement is necessary for the normal development of muscles and joints (see also Moessinger, this volume). This result also suggests that the precision of fit between the components of ball and socket joints is the result of a sculpting process produced by the constant movement of the joint while it is being formed.

At a more reductionistic level, the activity of motoneurons influences the differentiation of different types of muscle. Adult vertebrates have slow-twitch and fast-twitch muscles that differ in contraction properties, morphology, biochemistry, and pattern of innervation. Slow-twitch muscles are important for the maintenance of posture; fast-twitch muscles are used for bursts of rapid movement. In both birds and mammals, the nerves innervating the embryonic muscle influence the expression of fast and slow muscle properties (Vrbova, Gordon & Jones, 1978). For example, the cross-innervation of fast muscles with nerves that typically innervate slow muscles, redirects differentiation such that the prospective fast muscles assume the properties of slow muscles and vice-versa. Synaptic activity and/or muscle contraction at the myoneural junction seems to be involved because the modification of such activity produces similar changes in muscle properties in the absence of cross-innervation.

NATURALLY OCCURRING MOTONEURON DEATH

The embryo is a complex and harmonious constellation of cells whose developmental fate is coordinated, and in some instances determined, through a network of relationships. These relationships exist at several levels. The previous section described how joint development and myogenesis are shaped by spontaneous activity at embryonic stages. The influence of spontaneous motility on the survival of motoneurons will now be offered as an example of how embryonic activity can shape both postnatal behavior and central nervous system structure. It is, also, another case of an embryonic process that has no postnatal counterpart.

During the course of vertebrate embryonic development, thousands of apparently normal spinal cord motoneurons start to develop and then die

(Hamburger and Oppenheim, 1982). This is an instance where an apparently regressive event, cell death, is involved in what is typically viewed as the progressive or additive process of development. (Another case is the death of cells in the interdigital spaces of the paddle-like primordia that form the embryonic hands and feet. The surviving cells develop into discrete fingers and toes.) In the chick embryo, 40−60% of motoneurons die during the first third of incubation. The proportion of motoneurons that die is controlled by the size of the target of innervation, skeletal muscle. The number of dying motoneurons can be manipulated by increasing or decreasing the size of skeletal muscle mass being innervated. Extirpation (removal) of a limb bud at early developmental stages results in the death of almost all of the limb-innervating motoneurons. The addition of an extra (supernumerary) limb-bud saves many of the motoneurons that normally would have died. These results are explained in terms of competition by motoneurons for limited muscle innervation sites or trophic agents (Hamburger and Oppenheim, 1982).

Synaptic activity has also been implicated in the regulation of motoneuron numbers (Pittman and Oppenheim, 1978, 1979). The presynaptic and postsynaptic blockade of neuromuscular transmission with curare and curare-like drugs during the period of normal motoneuron death prevents almost all motoneuron loss. In a complementary study, the increase of neuromuscular activity by the direct electrical stimulation of peripheral nerves and limb muscles enhances motoneuron loss (Oppenheim and Nunez, 1982).

OUTSIDE-IN NEURAL AND BEHAVIORAL EVOLUTION: THE CENTRIPETAL HYPOTHESIS

The finding that the number of spinal cord motoneurons can be increased or decreased by experimentally altering muscle mass has some previously unappreciated ramifications for directing the course, increasing the precision, and accelerating the rate of behavioral evolution (Provine, 1984). The centripetal hypothesis of neurobehavioral evolution presented here involves an interaction between ontogenetic and phylogenetic processes.

Traditional accounts of neurobehavioral evolution assume that natural selection winnows behavioral variants produced by the spontaneous, random mutation of the nervous system. The possessor of a rare, successful mutation would enjoy the differential reproductive success that defines adaptive behavior. Since most mutations are presumed random, a process of behavioral evolution relying upon them must be slow, nonspecific and inefficient. In the proposed centripetal, outside-in process, the environment would select for or against muscle, the organ of locomotion; changes in the organization of the central nervous system would follow. Such a muscle oriented process is precise, rapid and efficient because natural selection acts directly upon the muscle to sculpt behavior.

The first step in understanding how the centripetal evolutionary process operates is to appreciate the dramatic transformations of muscle resulting from natural and artificial selection. Artificial selection by the modern animal husbandry industry has produced rapid increases in the muscle mass of meat animals. The heavy physique of beef cattle and massive pectoral muscles of meat chickens contrast with the much leaner ancestral forms. There has been no equivalent effort to select against muscle mass, but there have been numerous instances of natural selection. For example, acquired flightlessness is relatively common and rapid in onset among flighted birds that live in permissive environments that do not require flight (Provine, 1984). An important consequence of flightlessness is the loss of pectoral muscle mass no longer required for flight. The whale and the snake, both of which evolved from terrestrial quadrupeds, lost much of their original locomotor apparatus, including the limb and associated musculature, during phylogeny (Romer, 1970). Powerful natural selection against unnecessary, heavy and energetically expensive muscle probably causes profound and rapid loss of muscle no longer required for a specific movement. Increases in the mass of muscles required for more powerful or rapid movements would occur if the behavior produced by the muscles proved adaptive.

Selecting for or against muscles has the secondary consequence of selecting for or against related motoneurons in the spinal cord. This occurs through the embryonic processes considered in the previous section. The number of motoneurons is adjusted during development to match the size of the peripheral muscle mass by an increase or decrease in how many die in competition for limited muscle innervation sites or trophic agents (Hamburger and Oppenheim, 1982). This process has been viewed as a biological buffer mechanism to insure adequate innervation of a site (Katz and Lasek, 1978). It also has other, more dramatic consequences for neurobehavioral evolution (Provine, 1984).

The embryological evidence suggests that increases or decreases in muscle mass that occur through natural selection would produce corresponding increases or decreases in the number of motoneurons that survive embryonic development. The secondary and tertiary consequences of the selection for or against motoneurons are of principal interest here. The interneurons that are the pattern-generating circuits for locomotor behavior may also be affected indirectly by a change in muscle mass because the resulting loss of motoneurons deprives them of their innervation targets. Interneurons probably compete for motoneurons just as motoneurons compete for muscles (Provine, 1984). Thus, interneurons that have lost their usual motoneurons may degenerate, remain intact without motor function, or form synapses with different motoneurons that control the movement of different muscles. A substantial increase in muscle mass, and associated motoneuron survival, would provide interneurons with additional potential innervation sites, some of which might be with novel motoneurons that control novel muscles. The latter consequence could also produce a new pattern of movement in a given muscle.

A preliminary test of one aspect of the centripetal hypothesis has involved the search for remnants of flight in the emu, ostrich, cassowary, and rhea, all of which are giant flightless birds of the ratite group that are thought to have evolved from flighted ancestors (Provine, 1984). The vestigial wings of these birds are powered by a very small pectoral muscle mass. The flat, raft-like (ratite) sternum of these flightless birds contrasts with the deeply keeled sternum that supports the massive pectoral apparatus of flighted birds. The meager pectoral apparatus of the ratites is almost certainly correlated with a small number of brachial spinal motoneurons that drive the wings. Although the brachial motoneurons count of ratites is unknown, the report by Kappers and colleagues (1936) of a small brachial cord enlargement of the flightless ostrich relative to that of flying birds is consistent with a relatively small number of such motoneurons. None of the ratites perform either the spontaneous or drop-evoked wing-flapping that is characteristic of flying birds (Provine, 1984). This behavioral evidence is consistent with the view that a centripetal chain reaction that began with pectoral muscle and its motoneurons may have influenced the interneurons that are pattern generators for wing-flapping. (Not all flightless birds are incapable of wing-flapping. Penguins, perhaps the best flyers of all, propel themselves through the dense aquatic medium with short, narrow wings that are powered by massive pectoral muscles. Penguins perform vigorous spontaneous, but no drop-evoked wing-flapping.)

Speculation about the fate of interneuronal spinal cord pattern generating circuits produces some interesting possibilities. For example, do the neural circuits for obsolete behavior degenerate, linger in an inactive state, or become components for new circuits? To what extent is our nervous system a collection of circuits for archaic motor patterns? The Babinski and grasp reflexes may be produced by such obsolete circuitry. These curious types of behavior can be elicited only in neonates and in victims of brain damage; they are suppressed at other times. Our central nervous system may contain the circuitry for many such movements. Archaic circuits or behavior may accumulate when they are not maladaptive and subject to strong selection pressure. Some circuits may be physically intact but behaviorally inactive due to inhibition or the loss of excitatory input or effector organs. The motor programs produced by quiescent circuitry may increase the library of potential behavior from which future motor scores may be composed. The challenge for the experimenter is to activate these latent circuits and to recognize and interpret their output. Lesions of the central nervous system, drugs, or electrical stimulation may be useful in activating lost motor programs.

CONCLUSION

Detailed observations of embryos assist us in distinguishing the natural priorities of the developing organism from the fads and sometimes inappropriate concerns of theory-driven scientific disciplines. The hypothetico-deductive method that has been an effective approach to a number of problems in the biobehavioral sciences does not help us to select which hypothesis to test or what is important to know. In our haste to test hypotheses, we often neglect subtle lessons that are only taught by the embryo. Some of the lessons in this essay may seem strange to students of postnatal behavior. For example, sensation, motivation, and learning, have little, if any, relevance to embryonic behavior during much of development. This poses a dilemma for developmental psychologists and others who define their discipline as the study of these processes. Such individuals must either declare the realm of the embryo to be irrelevant, a common practice, or broaden their discipline to include the development of behavior, whatever its cause. This essay supports the second option. William Preyer (Gottlieb, 1973), a founder of the study of behavior development, appreciated the broad scope of developmental problems and led by example. Over a century ago, Preyer published what he considered to be two companion volumes. One was about behavioral embryology (Preyer, 1885); the other was devoted to child development (Preyer, 1882). The present concern with the uniqueness of embryos does not violate this ecumenical spirit; it is an attempt to redress an historical neglect of the prenatal period. Embryology is a rich source of facts, methods, and theory about ontogenetic and phylogenetic processes that is virtually unknown to students of postnatal behavior. The challenge of embryology, especially neuroembryology, should be accepted by students of behavior development.

Acknowledgements

The author's research has been supported by grant HD 11973 from the National Institute of Child Health and Human Development and by grants MH 28476 and MH 36474 from the National Institute of Mental Health.

References

Bekoff, A. (1976). Ontogeny of leg motor output in the chick embryo: A neural analysis. *Brain Research, 106*, 271–291.

Blakemore, C., & Cooper, G. F. (1970). Development of the brain depends on the visual environment. *Nature, 228*, 477–478.

Coghill, G. E. (1929). *Anatomy and the problem of behavior*. Cambridge: Cambridge University Press.

Drachman, D. B., & Sokoloff, L. (1966). The role of movement in embryonic joint development. *Developmental Biology, 14*, 401–420.

Gottlieb, G. (1973). Dedication to W. Preyer (1841–1897). In G. Gottlieb (Ed.), *Behavioral embryology* (pp. xv-xix). New York: Academic Press.

Grillner, S. (1975). Locomotion in vertebrates: Central mechanisms and reflex interaction. *Physiological Review, 55*, 247–304.

Haverkamp, L. (1986). Anatomical and physiological development of *Xenopus* embryonic motor system in the absence of neural activity. *Journal of Neuroscience, 6*, 1332–1337.

Haverkamp, L., & Oppenheim, R. W. (1986). Behavioral development in the absence of neural activity: Effects of chronic immobilization on amphibian embryos. *Journal of Neuroscience, 6*, 1138–1348.

Hamburger, V. (1963). Some aspects of the embryology of behavior. *Quarterly Review of Biology, 38*, 342–365.

Hamburger, V., & Oppenheim, R. W. (1982). Naturally occurring neuronal death in vertebrates. *Neuroscience Commentaries, 1*, 39–55.

Hamburger, V., Wenger, E., & Oppenheim, R. W. (1966). Motility in the chick embryo in the absence of sensory input. *Journal of Experimental Zoology, 162*, 133–160.

Hubel, D. H., & Wiesel, T. N. (1970). The period of susceptibility to the physiological effects of unilateral eye closure in kittens. *Journal of Physiology, 206*, 419–436.

Kappers, C. V. A., Huber, C. G., & Crosby, E. C. (1936). *Comparative anatomy of the nervous system of vertebrates, including man*. New York: Macmillan (reprinted by Hafner, New York, 1960).

Katz, M. J., & Lasek, R. J. (1978). Evolution of the nervous system: Role of ontogenetic buffer mechanisms in the evolution of matching populations. *Proceedings of the National Academy of Sciences, 75*, 263–288.

Landmesser, L. T., & O'Donovan, M. J. (1984). Activation patterns of embryonic chick hind limb muscles recorded *in ovo* and in an isolated spinal cord preparation. *Journal of Physiology, 347*, 189–204.

O'Donovan, M. J. & Landmesser, L. (1987). The development of hindlimb motor activity studied in the isolated spinal cord of the chick embryo. *Journal of Neuroscience, 7*, 3256–3264.

Oppenheim, R. W. (1981). Ontogenetic adaptations and retrogressive processes in the development of the nervous system and behavior: A neuroembryological perspective. In K. Connoly & H. F. R. Prechtl (Eds.), *Maturation and development: Biological and psychobiological perspective* (pp. 73–109).

Oppenheim, R. W., & Nunez, R. (1982). Electrical stimulation of hindlimb increases neuronal cell death in chick embryos. *Nature, 295*, 57–59.

Pittman, R., & Oppenheim, R. W. (1978). Neuromuscular blockade increases motoneuron survival during normal cell death in the chick embryo. *Nature, 271,* 364–366.

Pittman, R., & Oppenheim, R. W. (1979). Cell death of motoneurons in chick embryo spinal cord: IV. Evidence that a functional neuromuscular interaction is involved in the regulation of naturally occurring cell death and the stabilization of synapses. *Journal of Comparative Neurology, 187,* 425–446.

Porter, R. J., Mattson, R. H., Ward, A. A., & Dam, M. (1984). *Advances in epileptology: The XVth Epilepsy International Symposium.* New York: Raven Press.

Preyer, W. (1885). *Specielle physiologie des embryo.* Leipzig: Grieben's Verlag.

Preyer, W. (1882). *Die seele des kindes.* Leipzig: Fernan. (Translated as *The mind of the child.* New York: Appleton, Vol. I, 1888; Vol. II, 1889).

Provine, R. R. (1971). Embryonic spinal cord: Synchrony and spatial distribution of polyneuronal burst discharges. *Brain Research, 29,* 155–158.

Provine, R. R. (1972). Ontogeny of bioelectric activity in the spinal cord of the chick embryo and its behavioral implications. *Brain Research, 41,* 365–378.

Provine, R. R. (1973). Neurophysiological aspects of behavior development in the chick embryo. In G. Gottlieb (Ed.), *Behavioral embryology* (pp. 77–102). New York: Academic Press.

Provine, R. R. (1984). Wing flapping during development and evolution. *American Scientist, 72,* 448–455.

Provine, R. R. (1986). Behavioral neuroembryology: Motor perspectives. In W. T. Greenough & J. Juraska (Eds.), *Developmental neuropsychobiology* (pp. 213–239). New York: Academic Press.

Provine, R. R., Sharma, S. C., Sandel, T. T., & Hamburger, V. (1970). Electrical activity in the spinal cord of the chick embryo *in situ. Proceedings of the National Academy of Sciences, U. S., 65,* 508–515.

Ripley, K. L., & Provine, R. R. (1972). Neural correlates of embryonic motility in the chick. *Brain Research, 45,* 127–134.

Romer, A. S. (1970). *The vertebrate body,* 4th ed. Philadelphia: Saunders.

Schwartzkroin, P. A., & Wheal, H. V. (1984). *Electrophysiology of epilepsy.* London: Academic Press.

Vrbova, G., Gordon, T., & Jones, R. (1978). *Nerve-muscle interaction.* London: Chapman and Hall.

Windle, W. F. (1940). *Physiology of the fetus.* Philadelphia: Saunders.

On Observing the Human Fetus

Jason C. Birnholz
Department of Diagnostic Radiology and Nuclear Medicine
Rush-Presbyterian-St. Luke's Medical Center
Chicago, Illinois

Among the greatest medical advances in this century is a near elimination of maternal mortality and a vast reduction in infant mortality. The societal consequences in general attitudes about childhood, child rights, family planning and organization, and parental education are permeative, irreversible, and progressive. The success of American neonatology in achieving survival of small premature infants, coupled with the immediate availability of high level services for most of the urban population, has served to focus increasing technical interest on prenatal development, particularly on the functional maturation of the cardiovascular, respiratory, and central nervous systems. During this same time, there has been progressive sophistication in the use of ultrasonic imaging for non-invasive evaluation of the fetus for a range of diagnostic applications. This essay will consider the some ways in which recent ultrasonic observations have improved understanding of fetal development as well as the research possibilities for extending knowledge in this area.

Conventional ultrasound images are cross-sectional with depth as one axis, referred to as a "B-mode" display from the original, international radar terminology. Acoustic pulses propagate through soft tissues at an average velocity of 1.54 km/s. Images are synthesized on a line-by-line basis, with data along lines representing backscatter events during transit of an individual pulse. Shortly after launching, these pulses are shaped like a daddy long-legs spider, with most of the energy concentrated in a flattened central disc about which there is a symmetrical arrangement of side lobes. Pulse dimensions, which govern resolution, are less than a millimeter. Nearly all devices used clinically repetitively scan a restricted field of view at a rate of a few thousand data lines per second, arranged into 28 or more image frames per second. The principal performance characteristics are *temporal resolution* (the smallest amplitude movement that can be perceived), *contrast resolution* (the distinction of a target from its background, necessary for selective identification of different tissues), and *spatial resolution* (the smallest structural details that are defined). Pulses are distorted as they propagate through tissue, and idealized "beams" are deflected in complex ways from refraction and diffraction effects. In practical terms, image quality will vary from case to case, i.e., better in slender mothers than in obese ones, better with a normal amount of amniotic fluid than either with oligohydrammios or with polyhydramnios, when the fetus may be quite far from the probe. Within these constraints, however, quite life-like images with details in the low millimeter size range (Figure 1) are generally possible (Birnholz & Farrell, 1984). Finally, it should be emphasized that since the image is cross-sectional, scan plane selection is of ultimate importance in any examination. Consequently, the skill, experience, interest, and effort of the examiner remain the basic determinants of study adequacy and of the ability to make precise observations of both normal and abnormal development.

Since detail resolution is in the millimeter range, developmental studies have tended to concentrate on the postembryonic period, employing

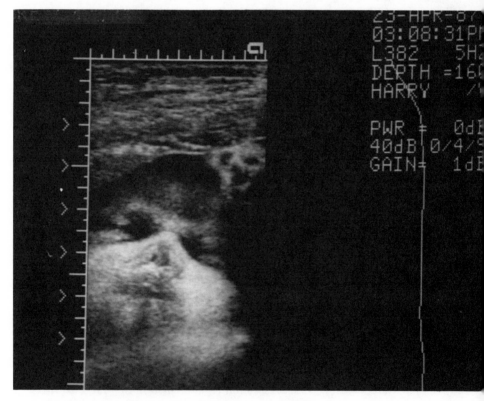

Figure 1. A frontal portrait of a well nourished mid third trimester male fetus (3.5 MHz, 80 mm aperture phased linear array; large scale markers in these images represent 10 mm tissue lengths).

the method in the first half of the first trimester for confirmation of intrauterine pregnancy and demonstration of fetal number or vitality. An operational assumption of biological safety is made for the method, which involves non-ionizing radiation exposure for which there will be no cumulative dose effects. The low energy and brief duty cycles of modern equipment appear to be far below the level necessary to produce cavitation or significant tissue heating. Moreover, in clinical practice with hand-held probes viewing well-vascularized areas, there is near constant tissue movement, on a wavelength scale, which prevents standing wave formation or similar forms of energy concentration. Some of the early devices emitted audible sounds in the 1000 to 3000 Hz range (from transducer excitation) and, occasionally, low frequency vibrations from servo-motors, which served to provoke fetal activity. This has been largely eliminated with the newer, electronic scanning instruments.

MOVEMENT

Movement, growth, and functional maturation are the basic attributes of post-embryonic fetal development. "Movement" refers to motor events observed ultrasonically, these being contraction of one or more anatomical muscle groups resulting in a gross displacement of some fetal part (Figure 2). Striated muscle fasiculations are usually not seen. Movement (e.g., non-muscular dynamics) also includes arterial pulsations, venous flows, and fluid in the upper respiratory tract (Figure 3). Cardiac movements are evident from 4 weeks conceptual age (CA), "simple" torso displacements are seen regularly by 5 weeks CA, and by 8 to 9 weeks there are already independent movements of either arm or leg. Muscle contractions may be spontaneous, peripherally originating events, but for the most part they are initiated (or suppressed) centrally.

Kicking in response to palpation was used as a sign of fetal well-being in the eighteenth century (Cazeau, 1871). Attention was drawn to spontaneous and evoked movements as a part of normal development by Preyer (1885) and others near the start of this century. Hooker (1952) and students attempted to define a developmental sequence of "fetal reflexes" from observations on previable infants in water baths, chiefly using tactile stimuli. Generalization of these innovative experiments was limited by test conditions of anoxia. Within a framework of "reflexes", there were proponents of a primitive "total body" response, which later differentiated, while others held with equal conviction that simple peripheral responses were combined into more complex, but still stereotyped, patterns

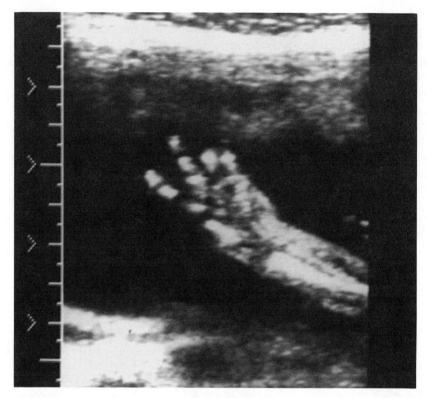

Figure 2. Ultrasound images are cross sectional. In this example, a 1/15 second duration scan is oriented to the fingers with are held in "victory" position. Motor behavior within a scan plane is assessed during visually continuous imaging.

over time. Little attention is now paid to these notions of reflex ontogeny, but emphasis is placed, instead, on central control and adaptability.

The fetus is visualized as a 3 to 5 mm long structure surmounting a larger yolk sac three to four weeks after conception. Heart rate is regular, but other movements are not then perceived. During the next two weeks the fetus becomes larger than the yolk sac and rests dependently within its amniotic bubble, presumably having a specific gravity very slightly greater than the surrounding fluid. By that time, simple extension-like movements of the upper spine are resolved, which tend to raise the fetus within the amnion, after which it settles slowly to a "rest" position. In another week, conjoint movements of the arms or legs are seen, and

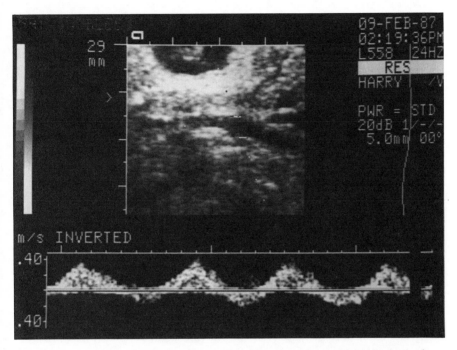

Figure 3. The Doppler sample volume (horizontal brackets) is placed within the trachea (upper insert, head left). The tracing plots flow velocity (m/s) against time (0.1 s markers), in this case showing chiefly retrograde fluid displacement in the upper airway. Intratracheal volume flow depends upon pump action of the diaphragm and valve effects of the larynx, glottis, and epiglottis. These are controlled centrally and become synchronized in the third trimester.

subsequently there is a rapid enlargement of the movement repertory, including isolated action of individual limbs. The abrupt increase in movement near the end of the first trimester illustrates a general observation about functional development: *maturation progresses as a nonlinear series of transitions* (probably involving threshold effects in cellular growth and biochemical diversity). A similar developmental pattern has been observed in a fetal rat model with continuous endoscopic monitoring (Smotherman & Robinson, 1986).

The rest position of the upper limbs early in the second trimester (when there is relatively abundant amniotic fluid) is a slight elevation of the arms and flaring of the elbows, flexion of the forearms, slight bending of the wrists, and flexion of the fingers. The hands are usually positioned at the level of the chin or shoulders. This position is reproduced exactly in astronauts sleeping under weightless conditions in space. Early second trimester forearm movements appear to be more or less random in timing and are abrupt in execution. When a hand strikes the face, there is an aversive reaction, with neck extension. Later, the neck flexion precedes forearm movement, facilitating hand-face contact. At a slightly later stage, there is persistent, exploratory-type hand-face contact that appears intentional, often associated with typical suckling movements of the lips, tongue, and jaw. Suckling is evoked by any cheek or lip contact. A portion of the finger or cord may be grasped by the lips; but thumbsucking itself is rare. The hand-face sequence illustrates a second general observation: *a broad range of individual physical movements are present relatively early, and their execution becomes smoother as they are coordinated into integrated patterns with time.*

Repetitive movements of the diaphragm (e.g., breathing) occur with moderate incidence from 12 to 16 weeks CA, then decline sharply until the start of the third trimester, after which they recur with progressive frequency and duration. Third trimester breathing patterns vary in their length, regularity and periodicity. These factors later stabilize into recurrent patterns associated with behavioral states (i.e., REM sleep, deep sleep and arousal; Prechtl, 1974). The third general observation is: *individual "permanent" motor sequences tend to appear, vanish, then recur in a modified, typically more "mature", version.* This sequence may represent primary central excitation, followed by development of specific forms of inhibition. Later, these active processes are melded into a balanced and controllable patterns (see also Smotherman & Robinson, this volume).

Early ultrasonic study of human fetal breathing movements suggested that late third trimester fetuses spend perhaps 20% of the time breathing and the remainder of the time in "apnea" (Patrick, Natale & Richardson, 1978). These observations are obviously at great variance with the norm for newborn infants at the same age. These early studies were flawed by a limiting definition of breathing as large amplitude movements of the chest wall and by poor spatial and temporal resolution of instruments then available. When diaphragm movements are evaluated directly, it is found that they occur at least 80% of the time late in the third trimester and their absence is likely due to central inhibition (Dawes et al., 1983). The incidence of breathing movements declines greatly with hypoxia as one of several, energy conserving, physiological compensations.

SOMATIC GROWTH

The type, timing, coordination, or modification of movement patterns already mentioned depend upon an anatomical substrate that increases in complexity during gestation. In terms of motoric capabilities, somatic growth may be compartmentalized into (a) the body, its appendages, and muscle groups, (b) neuronal and glial development of the central nervous system (including the pattern of their interconnections), and (c) sensors and their interaction with effectors through multi-element circuits. "Growth" is a global term that, for analysis, must be defined specifically for each individual part. This involves linear measurement of the body, calculation of fetal volume, and estimation of weight, assuming relatively little variation in specific gravity during normal gestation (Birnholz, 1986a). Weight increase is almost linear in the third trimester, with average values within plus or minus 10% of 1100 g at 28 weeks gestational age, 2200 g at 34 weeks, and 3300 g at 40 weeks (term) (Dunn, 1981).

There is remarkable consistency in somatic growth, at least through the midpoint of gestation. This consistency crosses ethnic, geographic and, probably, nutritional boundaries. Consistency underlies the ability to stage fetuses accurately from somatic measurements in the second trimester. Non-pathologic, genetic and acquired factors leading to differences in size or proportions at birth do not usually become manifest until the third trimester. A presumption is that developmental insults operating during the beginning of the first trimester result in malformations of one or more organs, and those in the early to mid second trimester result in profound, probably irreversible functional deficits that appear postnatally.

Cortical thickness in the motor strip areas (from the edge of lateral ventricle to the mantle peripherally) has been measured in the second trimester. A rapid increase in thickness occurs from about 12 to 14.5 weeks CA, plateaus until about 16 weeks, and exhibits a larger increase in thickness subsequently. These changes are believed to correspond to primary neuronal proliferation, neuronal migration, and glial proliferation (Sidman & Rakic, 1973). A delay has been observed in the onset of neuronal proliferation with trisomy-21 and some other conditions associated with mental retardation (Birnholz, 1986b). Neuronal migration continues throughout development. It recently has been suggested that impairment in migration accounts for the late sequellae of perinatal anoxic injury (Sarnat, 1987).

One of the outstanding features of brain growth in the third trimester is a marked increased in surface area of the cerebral cortex with sulcation (Figure 4). This process is also discontinuous with at least three phases of obvious change in surface pattern. Some features of surface development

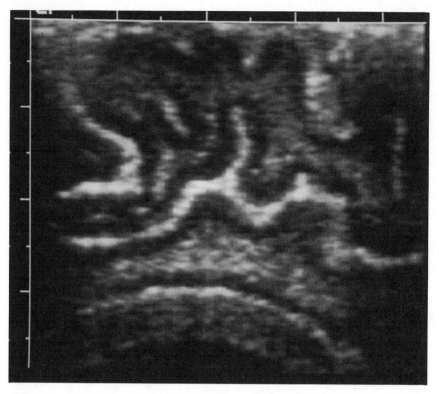

Figure 4. Magnification view of the right cingulate sulcus. Sulci appear white, gyri in gray with the peripheral rims corresponding to patterns of myelination.

of the cerebrum and cerebellum can be observed ultrasonically in the third trimester, although there is as yet no standardized method for quantifying these findings with cross-sectional imaging. Delays in sulcation are observed with trisomy-21 and with fetal alcohol syndrome; absence of sulcation diagnoses lissencephaly.

Slight degrees of lateral ventricular asymmetry may be seen at the start of the third trimester, but there is as yet no correlative data relating this feature (or gyral asymmetry) with handedness, general activity, or other facets of postnatal neuromotor behavior. Hand preference is expressed in infancy, but comparable prenatal observations have not been made, nor have pre-ultrasound suggestions about preferential fetal position and handedness (Michel, 1981) been confirmed.

SENSORY DEVELOPMENT

This discussion has already alluded to a conceptual overemphasis on reflex mechanisms during the first half of this century, evolving into a scheme of motor primacy. There is increasing documentation that fetal behavior becomes interactive environmentally as gestation progresses (see Fifer & Moon; Reppert & Weaver, this volume). Basic unresolved issues are what sensory stimuli, if any, are required for inducing development or for facilitating patterns that are already present.

The intrauterine environment is noisy with background intensity somewhere in the 50 to 80 dB range (Bench, 1968). The noise is a composite from the maternal gastrointestinal tract, from blood flow in larger arteries and, possibly, from airflow in the respiratory tree. Maternal voice seems to be particularly well transmitted into the uterus (Vince et al., 1985; see also Fifer & Moon, this volume). Sudden noises above background intensity prompt startle reactions in about 50% of fetuses at 24 weeks and all fetuses by 28 weeks (Birnholz & Benacerraf, 1983). Responses between 20 and 24 weeks have a noticeable latency, while by 28 weeks latency is on the order of a few tenths of a second. The startle, which includes forceful eye blinking, involves brain stem level circuitry that has been mapped thoroughly in experimental animals (Eaton, 1984).

It is possible to use ultrasound to study a range of individual facial movements (Figure 5) occurring spontaneously or prompted by complex auditory stimuli, such as voice and music. Early studies of auditory response used, of necessity, heart rate change as an endpoint for analysis (Bernard & Sontag, 1947), although it is not clear whether such observations provide physiologically unambiguous data. Studies of motor responses to repetitive, identical stimuli (Birnholz, 1984) have found decremental response in limb and torso components of the startle after 28 weeks CA. The number of pulses to extinction seems to decline exponentially with gestational age. This effect resembles a primitive form of habituation, and it is similar, if not identical, to sleep induction in a newborn infant by sensory overload (Brazelton, 1979). These decremental responses are due to subcortical mechanisms, as they have been observed in some cases of anencephaly (Graham, Leaviti & Stock, 1978). Capability for learning by the newborn infant is reviewed by Lipsitt (1977). However, it has been suggested that antenatal familiarization with maternal voice patterns influences postnatal perception (Spence & DeCasper, 1987).

There is less data concerning functional development of other sensory systems. Eye blinks can be elicited by bright light sources applied to the maternal lower abdomen late in the third trimester after auditory stimulation has placed the fetus in an alert state. Tactile sensation presumably

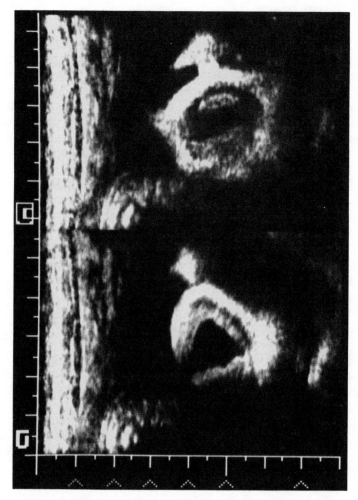

Figure 5. Sequential frontal views of the mouth at 31 weeks gestational age.

is the first to appear, particularly around the mouth. Inadvertent skin contact during amniocentesis provokes an aversive reaction in the third trimester but not in the second. There is some information on development of olfaction in an experimental animal model, and there is some limited data to the effect that fetal swallowing increases when sweet tasting solutions are infused into amniotic fluids (DeSnoo, 1937). Sensory organs and afferent pathways of different sensory systems can be identified early, but functional competence as indicated by motor end points involves not only the completion of neural circuitry but perception of a sensory event as distinct from neural background.

The final general observation is one of *continuity between fetal and infant behavior* (Prechtl & O'Brien, 1982; see also Smotherman & Robinson, this volume). This hardly seems to merit emphasis, but for the common assumption during the first half of this century that the fetus is an intra-uterine passenger, generally passive, with only limited capability for stereo-typed, reflex behavior. The scantiness of that outlook has become apparent from ultrasonic observations in utero and direct examination of surviving, small, premature infants. There is a wealth of behavioral variation and physiological compensation that occurs antenatally (Figure 6).

In this context, the question arises of whether or not a fetus cries in utero. Newborn infants begin to cry after the first few breaths, so that by

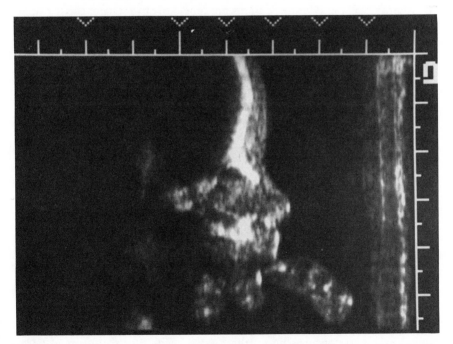

Figure 6. Profile view with the edge of the hand (lower right) contacting the lips. Most lip contacts evoke sucking movements. Thumbsucking is a postnatal behavior, occurring acciden-tally, and infrequently, in fetal life.

the principle of continuity, the later third trimester fetus certainly has this capability. Ultrasonic observation of expressive facial movements has already been noted, these comparing quite well with classic obervations on newborn infants. During the first few weeks of life, the infant spends anywhere from 50 to 150 minutes crying per day, the amount depending upon the level of nurturing and care (Aldrich et al., 1946). Crying is evoked by painful sensations, including hunger. Given the consistency of the intrauterine environment, including continuous nutritional and respiratory support via the placenta, one may conclude that the fetus can cry, but rarely does so unless provoked by some abrupt noxious stimulus, such as sharp needle contact during amniocentesis (particularly as performed prior to the availability of ultrasonic guidance).

A final concern in terms of behavioral integrity might be the question of fetal personality, which is the way that an individual fetus, or infant, interacts with less startling, but novel, stimuli in its environment. Some infants perform a great deal of spontaneous motor activity, while others are quieter. Some tend to be irritable, others are more phlegmatic. Some appear to be inquisitive, while others appear less interested in their environment. These types of features are amenable to prenatal classification with ultrasound, although this has not yet been accomplished in a systematic way. There has been some attempt to grade behavioral state transitions in the third trimester (Nijhuis et al., 1982), an approach which can be extended greatly with more detailed classification schemes possible with the current level of ultrasound equipment. Inasmuch as guided amniocentesis with small bore needles has become an essentially risk free procedure, there are responsibilities for exacting studies of fetal behavior, including visual stimulation through fiberoptic light sources and correlative monitoring of intrauterine pressure, vibration, sound, temperature, or amniotic fluid composition.

Dennis (1985), in her review article on fetal and child psychology, quotes pioneer W. Preyer:

"For thousands of years children have been born and lovingly tended and watched by their mothers, and for thousands of years learned men have disputed over the mental growth of the child, without even studying the children. As a rule, the experimental physiologist seldom visits the nursery, even when he is a father."

Ultrasonic imaging provides a unique, noninvasive means of extending our present understanding of infant development into the fetal period. As we have progressed from basic issues such as survival of the small premature human infant to concerns about the quality of its life, so too may these fetal studies contribute ultimately to techniques of optimizing human development and contribution, perhaps through "enriching" the fetal environment (Smotherman & Robinson, 1987).

References

Aldrich, C. A., Norval, M. A., Knop, C., & Venegas, F. (1946). The crying newly born babies. *Journal of Pediatrics*, *28*, 665–670.

Bench, J. (1968). Sound transmission to the human foetus through the maternal abdominal wall. *Journal of Genetic Psychology*, *113*, 85–87.

Bernard, J., & Sontag, L. W. (1947). Fetal reactivity to tonal stimulation: a preliminary report. *Journal of Genetic Psychology*, *70*, 205–210.

Birnholz, J. C. (1984). Fetal neurology. In R. Saunders & M. Hill, (Eds.), *Ultrasound Annual*, (pp. 139–160). New York: Raven Press.

Birnholz, J. C. (1986a). An algorithmic approach to accurate ultrasonic fetal weight estimation. *Investigative in Radiology*, *21*, 571–576.

Birnholz, J. C. (1986b). Ultrasonic studies of human fetal brain development. *Trends in Neuroscience*, *7*, 329–333.

Birnholz, J. C., & Benacerraf, B. R. (1983). The development of human fetal hearing. *Science*, *222*, 516–518.

Birnholz, J. C., & Farrell, E. E. (1984). Ultrasound images of human fetal development. *American Scientist*, *72*, 608–613.

Brazelton, T. B. (1979). Behavioral competence of the newborn infant. *Seminars in Perinatology*, *3*, 35–44.

Cazeau, P. (1871). A theoretic and practical treatise on midwifery (American edition, ed. W. R. Bullock). Philadelphia: Lindsay & Balkison.

Dawes, G. S., Gardner, W. N., Johnston, B. M., & Walker, D. W. (1983). Breathing in fetal lambs: the effect of brain stem section. *Journal of Physiology* (London), *355*, 533–553.

Dennis, M. (1985). William Preyer (1841–1897) and his neuropsychology of language acquisition. *Developmental Neuropsychology*, *1*, 287–315.

De Snoo, K. (1937). Das trinkende Kind im Uterus. *Monatsschrift fur Geburtshilfe und Gynaekologie*, *105*, 88–97.

Dunn, P. M. (1981). Variations in fetal growth: some causes and effects. In F. A. van Assche, & W. B. Robertson, (Eds.), *Fetal growth retardation*, (pp. 79–89). Edinburgh: Churchill Livingstone.

Eaton, R. C. (1984). *Neural mechanisms of startle behavior*. New York: Plenum Press.

Graham, F. H., Leaviti, L. A., & Stock, B. D. (1978). Precocious cardiac orienting in a human anencephalic infant. *Science*, *199*, 322–324.

Hooker, D. (1952). *The prenatal origin of behavior*. 18th Porter Lecture Series. Laurence: University of Kansas Press.

Lipsitt, L. P. (1977). The study of sensory and learning processes of the newborn. *Clinical Perinatology*, *4*, 163–186.

Michel, G. (1981). Right-handedness: a consequence of infant supine head-orientation preference? *Science*, *212*, 685–687.

Nijhuis, J. G., Prechtl, H. F. R., Martin, C. B., Jr., & Bots, R. S. G. M. (1982). Are there behavioural states in the human fetus? *Early Human Development*, *6*, 177–195.

60 J.C. Birnholz

Patrick, J., Natale, R., & Richardson, B. (1978). Patterns of human fetal breathing activity at 34 to 35 weeks' gestational age. *American Journal of Obstetrics and Gynecology, 132,* 507−513.

Prechtl, H. F. R. (1974). The behavioural states of the newborn infant (a review). *Brain Research, 76,* 185−212.

Prechtl, H. F. R., & O'Brien, M. J. (1982). Behavioural states of the full-term newborn. The emergence of a concept. In P. Stratton, (Ed.), *Psychobiology of the human newborn,* (pp. 53−73). New York: Wiley.

Preyer, W. (1885). *Spezielle Physiologie des Embryo.* Leipzig: Grieben.

Sarnat, H. B. (1987). Disturbances of late neuronal migrations in the perinatal period. *American Journal of Diseases of Children, 141,* 969−980.

Sidman, R. L., & Rakic, P. (1973). Neuronal migration with special reference to developing human brain: a review. *Brain Research, 62,* 1−35.

Smotherman, W. P., & Robinson, S. R. (1986). A method for endoscopic visualization of rat fetuses in situ. *Physiology & Behavior, 37,* 663−665.

Smotherman, W. P., & Robinson, S. R. (1987). Prenatal influences on development: behavior is not a trivial aspect of fetal life. *Developmental & Behavioral Pediatrics, 8,* 171−176.

Spence, M. J., & DeCasper, A. J. (1987). Prenatal experience with low-frequency maternal-voice sounds influence neonatal perception of maternal voice samples. *Infant Behavior & Development, 10,* 133−142.

Vince, M. A., Billing, A. E., Baldwin, B. A., Toner, J. N., & Weller, C. (1985). Maternal vocalisations and other sound in the fetal lamb's sound environment. *Early Human Development, 11,* 179−190.

BEHAVIORAL ORGANIZATION

Pattern Construction in Behavior

John C. Fentress and Peter J. McLeod

Departments of Psychology and Biology
Dalhousie University
Halifax, Nova Scotia
Canada

In this chapter we survey some basic conceptual issues in behavioral development. Descriptions of behavioral patterning, the antecedents of these patterns, and the roles of experience in the development of behavior patterns are each points we consider. Although our own work has concentrated upon postnatal patterns of behavioral expressions, the issues we address are also relevant to fetal behavior. With respect to the processes involved in the development of patterned action, we see no obvious reason to form a hard dichotomy between prenatal and postnatal periods, even though they have most often been studied separately (cf. Prechtl, 1984; Greenough, Black & Wallace, 1987; Smotherman & Robinson, 1987).

How patterns are constructed, the primary issue we address, is a ubiquitous problem in both behavioral and biological science (e.g., Ede, 1978; Fentress & McLeod, 1986). Patterns involve separable events that are also connected together in space and time. The crucial question for analysis is how these separations and combinations co-occur during development (Fentress, in press). The rules by which events undergo the complementary processes of separation and combination during the development, however, are not well understood. We argue that this is in part a problem of how we describe behavior.

THE PROBLEM OF BEHAVIORAL TAXONOMY

Integrated behavior patterns are among the basic products of biology upon which natural selection has its most direct impact (Darwin, 1872). That there are separations among classified behavioral events is non-controversial, nor is it controversial that such separated events combine together in space and time. It is relative separation that defines both biological and behavioral patterns in their most basic sense.

When, and by what criteria, do we say that one behavioral event is

63

separable from another? This question reflects most problems of order and co-order in the life sciences (Fentress, 1986, in press). Individually defined mouse grooming strokes, or wolf displays, or properties of human speech must be separable to be effective. Yet such isolated properties of behavior are more or less intimately connected during functional expressions (e.g., wolf displays, McLeod, 1987). In human speech there are similar intimate connections between the detailed forms of individual articulations (Studdert-Kennedy, 1981).

Hierarchical Models and Their Limits

One method of addressing this problem is to arrange behavioral events in a hierarchical manner. As illustration, individually abstracted components of mouse grooming are repeated in several distinct groupings, rather as are letters that comprise words in a phrase (Fentress, 1972). However, stress and timing events that contribute to a defined motor action can also permeate the expression of a number of actions (Fentress, in press; Kelso, 1986; Rosenbaum, 1985). Whether stress or timing events should thus be viewed as "lower" or "higher" than the abstracted actions to which they contribute is thus moot. The apparent hierarchical organization of patterned behavior varies with the chosen methods of analysis (Fentress, in press).

Traditional hierarchical concepts include alternative criteria, such as whether "higher" regions "issue commands" or participate in more "democratic conversations" with their subcomponents (e.g., through the prevalent existence of re-entrant loops in most neural systems, parallel as well as sequential control parameters, etc.; Fentress, in press). Most hierarchical models employed in behavior and biology today also remain essentially static, which can obscure rather than clarify organizational dynamics (cf., Kelso, 1986). Throughout the development of behavioral expression organisms must deal with problems that involve dynamic principles of "co-ordering" among body parts, the body's orientation in the external world, etc.

From Descriptions to Models of Developmental Control

Golani and Fentress (1985) found that descriptions of individual limb segment kinematics, forepaw trajectories, and contacts between the forelimbs and the face in mice provide separable insights into ontogenetic change.

Variables such as timing or amplitude of movement can also cross descriptive categories, and thereby provide useful insights. In a recent study of rat exploration, Eilam and Golani (in press) demonstrated how abstracted movement properties such as lateral, foreward and vertical movements can yield systematic ontogenetic progressions. Even basic questions about behavioral stereotypy and direction of ontogenetic change can be influenced by one's measures (e.g. Golani and Fentress, 1985; Fentress, in press).

The relative nature of connections and separations among behavioral properties has important implications for our views about development. For example, it may prove important to ask if developmental changes in the temporal patterning of one behavioral event will have ramifications for the timing of another related behavioral event. The potential interest in such questions can be seen in the recent demonstration by Keele and Ivry (1987) that cerebellar disorders in humans can affect the precision of timing in both motor performance and perception. How might modalities interact in the construction and performance of patterned actions?

With respect to the neurobiological substrates of developing systems in perception, both synergistic and competitive interactions can be seen across modalities. Thus, Knudsen and Knudsen (1985) found that visual experience in barn owls is important to the directional turning of auditory cues, and Rauschecker (1984) found an increased responsiveness of neurons in the superior colliculus to auditory stimuli in cats that had been visually deprived. At the level of movement patterns, data are much less clear. However, one might expect that developmental changes in one parameter of movement will have ramifications that extend both to that movement used in novel contexts, and to other movement parameters.

Such considerations lead to the fundamental question of where basic commonalities and separations are for the systems that contribute to behavior throughout ontogeny. How do we draw the boundaries that separate one property of behavior from another so that their rules of interconnection can also be clarified? For studies of ontogeny, both the boundaries that isolate one "system" from another, and the rules that join these systems together, are in a state of flux. It is thus often difficult to know where to anchor one's observations.

Dynamic Control Systems As "Centers" with "Surrounds"

One can address many of these problems by conceptualizing both integrative and developmental control systems as multidimensional, and with a dynamic balance between "core" states of activation and larger fields of protective "inhibitory" surround (Fentress, 1984, in press). As illustration, in many sensory systems pathways appear to operate on a center-surround basis, which can be defined at complementary levels of organization (e.g., Konishi, 1986).

A frequent feature of behavioral control systems is that lateral inhibition networks have a higher threshold for expression than do central excitatory cores. One consequence, discussed by Fentress (1984, in press), is that very early or very late, and/or weak patterns of activation may have comparatively broad consequences in behavioral pattern construction, often exhibited by a facilitation of ongoing state. Strongly activated systems are more focussed, and more likely to respecify ongoing states. Analogous models may apply to development (see below; and Fentress, in press).

EXPERIENCE AND BOUNDARIES IN BEHAVIOR PATTERN CONSTRUCTION

Most models of morphological embryology start from the premise that early stages of organization are relatively diffuse. Processes of differentiation play major roles. A complementary issue emphasized in the ethological literature is how differentiated events become combined into higher-order functional ensembles (Fentress and McLeod, 1986; Thelen, 1986; see also Thelen; Robinson & Smotherman, this volume). Separable aspects of behavioral expression often achieve function through associations with other action properties.

An initial question for behavioral embryology is what aspects of behavioral expression any feature of experience should influence. A second question is how the ramifications of any experience permeate other patterns. A third question is how experiential ramifications are expressed in different behavioral contexts. Each of these questions is analogous to problems of integration in behavioral performance more generally.

Dichotomous Roles of Experience

To what extent do we expect environmental events to provide simple "instructions" reflected isomorphically by future behavior? Might experience during development play more diverse roles? Greenough and coworkers (1987) have recently suggested the value of making a distinction between "*experience-expectant*" and "*experience-dependent*" events during development. This distinction refers to how certain experiences normally reflect an organism's species-characteristic environment, while others are more unique. A related distinction is between experiences that "select" among preexisting pathways versus "instruct" novel developmental pathways (e.g., Edelman & Finkel, 1984).

It is not always clear whether "expectant" versus "dependent" or "selectional" versus "instructional" sources of information during ontogeny will have similar properties of generalization. Often it is difficult to know where to draw the boundaries between these two sets of polarities. However, the point that there may be quite different consequences as well as routes of experience deserves further investigation.

The only way such questions can be explored is to separate properties of behavioral expression from one another, and then see how these interact. Relative buffers from experience are as important as sensitiveness to experience. For example, McLeod (1987) has provided evidence that the basic performance patterns of wolf social communication displays may be less dependent upon details of experience than are the responses to these displays. This perspective fits well with the general idea of retrograde development in behavior, in which basic motor patterns appear less dependent upon particular routes of experience than are their sensory/perceptual precursors in adult life (e.g., review by Fentress & McLeod, 1986). However, even the differentiation of muscle reflects "experiences" provided by the nerves that contact them (see review by Purves & Lichtman, 1985).

Boundaries of Developmental Change

Early rules of connectivity cross many of the boundaries that initial taxonomies might suggest to be impermeable. For example, Stanfield and coworkers (1982) found in newborn rats that many neurons from the occipital ("visual") cortex project to the pyramidal ("motor") tract. Through apparent processes of subsequent terminal retraction these early projections are eliminated. Such observations lead to many fascinating but as yet unexplored questions, such as whether early "diffuse" sensori-motor connections have developmental relevance, and whether experiential manipulations during development can clarify the extent and limits of this relevance.

Rebillard and coworkers (1977, 1980) found that during early postnatal ontogeny in kittens, the auditory cortex responds to a variety of modalities (e.g., to visual as well as to auditory inputs). This polysensory convergence becomes restricted during maturity, but this restriction of responsiveness to non-auditory inputs can be reduced considerably by surgical removal of the cochlea (thus eliminating normal auditory input). At the behavioral level, Spear and Molina (1987) have recently offered arguments in favor of early "amodal" consequences of experience, which also tend to become restricted and specialized with age. Motivational processes may also appear to have less clear boundaries early in development, with the result that the direction on animal's behavior takes is determined in part by such factors as body posture (e.g., sensori-motor "traps"; Fentress, 1984, in press).

There are many mechanisms that underlie this commonly observed progressive restriction, such as the elimination of individual neurons and connections among neurons (Purves & Lichtman, 1985; see also Provine, this volume). Much of this appears due to competitive interactions, where neighboring populations of cellular events succeed at the expense of others. Possible synergistic relations among developmental events also deserve consideration, although here the available data are at present inadequate for any broad generalisations to be drawn (see above).

An illustration of competitive interactions in the restriction of neuronal projections is seen in the work by Constantine-Patton and Law (1978) on the frog visual system. In mammals, the two eyes project to each visual cortex, with the result that during development alternating "bands" of projections for the two eyes can be observed. Monocular visual deprivation prevents the formation of this banding pattern, due to the elimination of normal competitive interactions between the eyes. In frogs, visual projections from each eye are restricted to the contralateral tectum, which thus does not exhibit this banding pattern. However, if a third eye is implanted into the central head region of a tadpole, axons from two eyes project to the same tectum. The result is that "ocular dominance columns" similar to those found in mammals are produced. Neuronal projections from the transplanted and normal eye compete for common territory, and thereby mutually restrict their fields of influence. Clearly, patterns of differentiation (restriction) represent populational events that can only be understood fully by taking into account the dynamic network of interactions that operate during ontogeny.

As a final illustration at the neuronal level, rats and other rodents develop specific projections from individual vibrissae to particular regions of the somatosensory cortex, which segregate through competitive interactions into receptive "barrels". When individual whiskers are cauterized during early postnatal development, their corresponding whisker barrels are reduced or eliminated, with concomitant spreading of neighboring barrels (Woolsey, Durham, Harris, Simons & Valentino, 1981). At present, there have been no systematic studies of the possible behavioral consequences (e.g., upon grooming) of such manipulations. Nor have there been any studies concerned with possible roles of feedback from early grooming movements (including prenatal movements; cf. Smotherman and Robinson, 1987) upon the differentiation of these barrels.

TOWARD EMBRYOLOGICAL MODELS OF BEHAVIORAL DEVELOPMENT

From the fertilized egg through blastula and gastrula stages into neurolation and beyond, the developing organism not only responds as a whole to its environment, but compartments that are being formed within the organism open and close routes of communication with their neighbors. The fundamental question is how developing systems attain intrinsic order through interactions with their surroundings (Fentress, in press). The basic mechanism is one of differential gene expression that in turn leads to the molding of higher-order phenotypic properties. However, as stated by Davidson (1986, p. 2) "causal links between genome and embryo remain largely undescribed".

We emphasize that references to gene activation and selection among potential gene products do not minimize the importance of experiential factors during development. Events of determination and subsequent differentiation are made possible only through differential experiences that play upon cells at very early developmental stages. Stent (1981) has similarly noted that simple genetic programming models for complex phenotypes are limited due to emerging phenotypic properties that also play against one another at a number of levels. Further, genes normally operate through pleiotrophic pathways distributed in space and time, and even relatively simple phenotypic characters are usually the result of multigenic contributions.

The differentiation of the vertebrate neural crest into such diverse cellular descendants as pigment cells, neurons and autonomic glia, etc., is illustrative of intrinsic/extrinsic relations that provide a useful conceptual framework for pattern construction more broadly (e.g., Weston, Ciment, & Girdlestone, 1984). Grafting experiments indicate that these different cellular products reflect the environments which migrating and genetically equivalent crest cells encounter. Experiments with mutant animals have clarified the interplay between events intrinsic to the migrating cells and their encounters with extracellular matrix macromolecules. Certain mutations are relatively autonomous in that their primary action is restricted to particular crest descendant cells, whereas other mutations are non-autonomous in the sense that they operate by changing environmental cues within which crest derived cells are embedded.

As a second example, derivative cells that make up the neurons of the autonomic system are of two basic types, adrenergic (sympathetic ganglion cells) and cholinergic (parasympathetic ganglion cells). Transplantation and tissue culture studies show that these differences in transmitter production reflect different experiential histories of neuronal precursor cells. Patterson and his colleagues (e.g., Patterson, 1978) followed individual neurons in environmentally controlled cultures. The cholinergic-adrenergic balance could be shifted through environmental manipulations, without changes in cell numbers (i.e., induction rather than selection). Contextual (environmental) events are important at all levels.

CONTEXTUAL FACTORS IN EXPRESSION

The importance of examining contextual variables in behavioral expression is illustrated by a study by Berridge and Fentress (1986). They showed that the consequences of lesions of afferent branches of the trigeminal nerve in adult rats depend upon the particular circumstances under which specific acts (e.g. grooming) are observed. For example, during relatively flexible phases of postprandial grooming these deafferentation procedures produced marked changes in the form of certain grooming movements that were, however, preserved during more rigorous and stereotyped phases of the same actions. A given change in developmental experience may similarly have either marked or minimal effects depending upon the circumstances under which behavior is observed.

McLeod (1987) provided evidence that in wolf social development it is imperative to examine individual actions within even broader contexts if one wishes to understand precursors of these actions (cf., Moran, Fentress & Golani, 1981; Havkin, 1981; Golani, 1976). For example, during ontogeny there appear to be different relative constraints on behavior that have an intrinsic basis, as defined by actions of the individual animal, and an extrinsic basis, as defined by actions of the social partner. Specific contextual factors were found to be relevant at one stage but not at either earlier or later stages (see Smotherman & Robinson, this volume).

A point we make is that all responses to ongoing behavioral states are a joint reflection of behavioral state and concurrent events. Thus, in the study of integrative performance it is important to know what an animal is doing or has recently been doing in measuring its response to particular extrinsic perturbations (Fentress, 1972). During development similar issues arise with respect to the effects of experience.

ON EVOLUTIONARY PERSPECTIVES IN DEVELOPMENT

Organisms are constructed through evolution to take advantage of a wide range of developmental events that may have diverse consequences. Attempts at formal modeling are presently at a very preliminary stage. One general approach that deserves further exploration at the behavioral level is that developing systems become refined through a combined process of autocatalysis "within" a given system, and inhibition "between" systems (Meinhardt, 1982). These two processes together can result in complex patterns of synergistic and antagonistic relations. Computer simulations from this perspective lead to complex patterns from initially homogenous beginnings, provided that one or another route of perturbation is introduced. From that point onward the developing systems become progressively "self-organized".

Of course, such general models must be supplemented with explicit considerations of particular routes and parameters of experience. Here the work of Gottlieb on vocal pattern recognition in ducklings is illustrative (e.g. Gottlieb, in press). Gottlieb isolated parameters of vocal patterning in several species of ducks, and then asked how exposure to these patterns during ontogeny might affect subsequent behavioral preferences. One of Gottlieb's most important findings is that even prenatal experience with species-characteristic distress calls can affect the subsequent preference of ducklings toward "assembly calls" of their species. This is noteworthy in that distress and assembly calls differ considerably from one another in their details of articulation. However, they also share important abstracted properties, such as rhythmic expression and the presence of descending tones, which indicates that the developing organism can often utilize such abstracted properties for the perfection of behavioral properties that may subserve quite different functional endpoints.

This leads to consideration of genetic predispositions in the light of developmental experience. Developmental processes reflect the evolutionary history of an organism. This implies the existence of biases to favor certain outcomes over others. As illustration, orientation specific cells in the visual cortex of cats normally show a bias toward greatest sensitivity to vertical and horizontal lines, rather than to lines along a diagonal. Leventhal and Hirsch (1975) report that early exposure to diagonal lines does not overcome this bias. There is even the suggestion that in contrast to visually deprived animals, animals exposed only to diagonal lines develop improved sensitivity to lines that are vertically and horizontally oriented. This is of considerable interest in that it indicates that the environment is not merely stamping orientation specificity on cells that are equipotential prior to visual experience. One might ask next whether facilitation of pre-existing developmental biases, such as noted here, operates at a different threshold than that for the respecification of these biases.

EXPERIENTIAL VARIANCE: MIGHT THRESHOLDS DETERMINE EFFECTS?

There are both buffers against and sensitivities to the effects of experiences normally encountered during ontogeny. One question that arises from this that has received relatively little attention concerns the consequences of incomplete or distorted experiences during development. We have no general rules for anticipating the effects of variation in "levels" or "properties" of experience.

One approach to this problem is to consider the possibility that moderate amounts of a wide range of experiences may have relatively broad influences, thus facilitating pre-existing developmental trends. Higher levels of "off target" experiences may be more likely to restructure the course of development (cf., Fentress, in press). The basic implication of this idea is that developmental processes are normally constrained. These constraints reflect previous phenotypic history. The possibility that organisms can utilize moderately degraded experiences of moderate intensity, or "fill-in" details from incomplete experience, offers exciting opportunities for future research.

The general importance of threshold considerations for problems of nervous system development has been addressed recently by Singer (1986). He argues convincingly that many events that activate integrative pathways can do so at a lower level of stimulation than events that respecify pre-existing structures. Horn (1985) has provided exciting recent evidence that the consequences of presenting chickens with abnormal models to follow can vary with the time frame of subsequent imprinting tests. In brief summary, Horn and his colleagues have found that the provision of a distorted model can enhance preferences for a normal model hours after this same exposure respecifies earlier measure preferences. Since many aspects of behavioral activation decline with time, one might indeed suggest that Horn and his colleagues have provided at least initial support for the dual threshold model noted above.

SOME FINAL COMMENTS ON THE NATURAL HISTORY OF BEHAVIORAL DEVELOPMENT

We have tried to emphasize the importance of careful and complementary descriptions of behavior, as well as careful and complementary views about underlying developmental processes. The descriptions imply that intact organisms operate through complex networks of separations and recombinations of individual events, with the result that the boundary distinguishing one category of behavior from another is often relative rather than absolute. Underlying developmental processes also exhibit still poorly understood separations and connections that are dynamically ordered, relational and multileveled (Fentress, 1986). Fundamental to future progress is the establishment of a more adequate base for evaluating how self-organizing processes also display sensitivities to their broader contexts of operation. We can expect sensitivities to particular extrinsic events to vary quantitatively, qualitatively and temporally in ways that normally assure the adaptive capabilities of the developing organism over each phase of its prenatal and postnatal life (cf. Alberts, 1987; Smotherman and Robinson, 1987).

An issue that we have not addressed is the ontogenetic origins of individual differences. These differences in performance capabilities, and strategies of their utilization, bring the study of development importantly back to considerations of natural selection. It is the relative capabilities and performance strategies of animals that accounts for their ultimate competitive status.

The distinction between capabilities and strategies can be useful in giving us future tools for thinking about development in more critical terms. Environments as well as organisms change during development (see Hofer, this volume). Actions that serve one function at one age may serve quite different functions at another age, and capabilities may develop prior to their usefulness in terms of overt behavior. Often these capabilities can be revealed through the provision of environmental supports, such as holding infant mice in an appropriate sitting posture to elicit grooming (Golani and Fentress, 1985) or providing human infants with the supports necessary to exhibit patterns of locomotory movements that are later involved in stepping (Thelen, 1986). A recent example of the establishment of developmental circuits before their normal utilization is provided by Eilam and Golani (in press). They showed that amphetamine injections in infant rats can lead to the appearance of movement capacities that are normally seen hours or days later.

There may be behavioral capabilities that develop before they show any functional consequence in themselves, yet the developmental events that underlie these capabilities may also contribute not only to future performance but also reflect the establishment of developmental pathways that have important immediate consequences. And of course the thorny issue of continuity versus discontinuity in development is now becoming recognized as one that reflects in part what measures we have assumed to be most important (e.g. Bekoff, 1981; Oppenheim, 1981; Prechtl, 1984; Alberts, 1987; Smotherman and Robinson, 1987; see also Smotherman & Robinson, this volume).

These brief considerations reflect how important it is to combine broad natural history perspectives with concurrent technical advances aimed at smaller subsets of issues. Often in the former case we must ask ourselves what questions we have not yet asked so that in the latter case we can learn how to ask these questions more precisely. This is obviously a very exciting time for studies of behavioral development across all time spans and levels of organization in diverse species.

Acknowledgements

Our thanks to Bill Smotherman and Scott Robinson for their invitation to participate in this volume, and for their constructive comments throughout. We also acknowledge the contributions of our many colleagues at Dalhousie, along with financial support from Graduate Studies at Dalhousie University, plus MRC and NSERC monies that have contributed significantly. W. Danilchuk helped with the final preparation of our manuscript.

References

Alberts, J. R. (1987). Early learning and ontogenetic adaptation. In N. A. Krasnegor, E. M. Blass, M. A. Hofer & W. P. Smotherman, (Eds.), *Perinatal development: a psychobiological perspective*, (pp. 11–37). Orlando: Academic Press.

Bekoff, A. (1981). Embryonic development of the neural circuitry underlying motor coordination. In W. M. Cowan, (Ed.), *Studies in developmental neurobiology*, (pp. 134–170). New York: Oxford University Press.

Berridge, K. C., & Fentress, J. C. (1986). Contextual control of trigeminal sensorimotor function. *Journal of Neuroscience, 6*, 325–330.

Constantine-Patton, M., & Law, M. I. (1978). Eye-specific termination bands in tecta of three-eyed frogs. *Science, 202*, 639–641.

Darwin, C. (1872). *The expression of the emotions in man and animals*. London: John Murray.

Davidson, E. H. (1986). *Gene activity in early development* (3rd edition). New York: Academic Press.

Edelman, G. M., & Finkel, L. H. (1984). Neuronal group selection in the cerebral cortex. In G. M. Edelman, W. E. Gall, & W. M. Cowan, (Eds.), *Dynamic aspects of neocortical function*, (pp. 653−695). New York: John Wiley & Sons.

Ede, D. A. (1978). *An introduction to developmental biology*. New York: John Wiley & Sons.

Eilam, D., & Golani, I. (in press). The ontogeny of exploratory behavior in the house rat (*Rattus rattus*): the immobility-mobility gradient. *Developmental Psychobiology*.

Fentress, J. C. (1972). Development and patterning of movement sequences in inbred mice. In J. Kiger, (Ed.), *The biology of behavior*, (pp. 38−132). Corvallis: Oregon State University Press.

Fentress, J. C. (1984). The development of coordination. *Journal of Motor Behavior, 16*, 99−134.

Fentress, J. C. (1986). Development of coordinated movement: dynamic, relational and multileveled perspective. In H. T. A. Whiting & M. C. Wade, (Eds.), *Motor development in children: aspects of coordination and control*, (pp. 77−105). Dordrecht: Martinus Nijhoff.

Fentress, J. C. (in press). Organizational patterns in action: local and global issues in action pattern formation. In [G. Edelman, W. E. Gall & W. M. Cowan, (Eds.)], *Signal and sense: local and global order in perceptual maps*. New York: John Wiley & Sons.

Fentress, J. C., & McLeod, P. (1986). Motor patterns in development. In E. M. Blass, (Ed.), *Handbook of behavioral neurobiology, vol. 8, Developmental psychobiology and developmental neurobiology*, (pp. 35−97). New York: Plenum.

Golani, I. (1976). Homeostatic motor processes in mammalian interactions: A choreography of display. In Perspectives in Ethology, Vol. 2, P. P. G. Bateson and P. H. Klopfer, eds., pp. 69−134, Plenum Press, New York.

Golani, I., and Fentress, J. C. (1985). Early ontogeny of face grooming in mice. *Developmental Psychobiology*, 18(6), 529−544.

Gottlieb, G. (in press) Development of species identification in ducklings: Malleability of species-specific perception. *Journal of Comparative Psychology*.

Greenough, W. T., J. E. Black, and C. S. Wallace (1987). Experience and brain development. *Child Development*, 58(3): 539−559.

Havkin, G. Z. (1981). Form and strategy of combative interactions between wolf pups (*Canis lupus*). Ph.D. Thesis, Dalhousie University, Halifax, Nova Scotia.

Horn, G. (1985). Memory, Imprinting, and the Brain: An Inquiry into Mechanisms, Clarendon Press, Oxford.

Keele, S. W., and R. I. Ivry (1987). Timing and force control: A modular analysis. IREX presentation, Soviet-American Bilateral Exchange Conference on Motor Control, Moscow.

Kelso, J. A. S. (1986). Pattern formation in speech and limb movements involving many degrees of freedom. *Exper. Brain Res. Series* 15: 105−128.

Knudsen, E. I., and P. F. Knudsen (1985). Vision guides the adjustment of auditory localization in young barn owls. Science, 230: 545−548.

Konishi, M. (1986). Centrally synthesized maps of sensory space. *Trends in Neuroscience*, 9: 163−168.

Leventhal, A. G., and H. V. B. Hirsch (1975). Cortical effect of early selective exposure to diagonal lines. *Science*, 190: 902−904.

McLeod, P. J. (1987). Aspects of the early social development of timber wolves (*Canis lupus*). Ph.D. Thesis, Dalhousie University, Halifax, Nova Scotia.

Meinhardt, H. (1982). Generation of structures in a developing organism. In *Developmental Order: Its Origin and Regulation*, pp. 439−461, Alan R. Liss, Inc., New York.

Moran, G., J. C. Fentress, and I. Golani (1981). A description of relational patterns during "ritualized fighting" in wolves. *Animal Behaviour*, 29: 1146–1165.

Oppenheim, R. W. (1981). Ontogenetic adaptations and retrogressive processes in the development of the nervous system and behavior. In Maturation and Behavior Development, K. Connolly and H. Prechtl, eds., pp. 73–109, Spastics Society Publications, London.

Patterson, P. H. (1978). Environmental determination of autonomic neurotransmitter functions. Ann. Rev. *Neuroscience*, 1: 1–17.

Prechtl, H. F. R. (1984). Continuity and change in early neural development. In *Continuity of Neural Functions from Prenatal to Postnatal Life*, H. F. R. Prechtl, ed., pp. 1–15, Blackwell Scientific, Oxford.

Purves, D., and J. W. Lichtman (1985). Principles of Neural Development, Sinauer Associates, Sunderland, Massachusetts.

Rauschecker, J. P. (1984). Neuronal mechanisms of developmental plasticity in the cat's visual system. *Human Neurobiology*, 3: 109–114.

Rebillard, G., M. Rebillard, and R. Pujol (1980). Factors affecting the recording of visual evoked potentials from the deaf cat primary cortex. *Brain Research* 188: 252–254.

Rebillad, G., E. Carlier, M. Rebillard, and R. Pujol (1977). Enhancement of visual responses on the primary auditory cortex of the cat after an early destruction of cochlear receptors. *Brain Research*, 129: 162–164.

Rosenbaum, D. A. (1985). Motor programming: A review and scheduling theory. In *Motor Behavior: Programming, Control and Acquisition*, H. Heuer, U. Kleinbeck, and K.-H. Schmidt, eds., pp. 1–33, Springer-Verlag, Berlin/Heidelberg/New York/Tokyo.

Singer, W. (1986). Neuronal activity as a shaping factor in postnatal development of visual cortex. In W. T. Greenough & J. M. Juraska, (Eds.), *Developmental Neuropsychobiology*, (pp. 271–293). Orlando: Academic Press.

Smotherman, W. P., & Robinson, S. R. (1987). Psychobiology of fetal experience in rat. In N. A. Krasnegor, E. M. Blass, M. A. Hofer, & W. P. Smotherman, (Eds.), *Perinatal development: a psychobiological perspective*, (pp. 39–60). Orlando: Academic Press.

Spear, N. E., & Molina, J. C. (1987). The role of sensory modality in the ontogeny of stimulus selection. In N. A. Krasnegor, E. M. Blass, M. A. Hofer, & W. P. Smotherman, (Eds.), *Perinatal development: a psychobiological perspective*, (pp. 83–110). Orlando: Academic Press.

Stanfield, B. B., O'Leary, D. D. M., & Fricks, C. (1982). Selective collateral elimination in early postnatal development restricts cortical distribution of rat pyramidal tract neurons. *Nature*, 298, 371–373.

Stent, G. S. (1981). Strength and weakness of the genetic approach to the development of the nervous system. *Annual Review Neuroscience*, 4, 163–194.

Studdert-Kennedy, M. (1981). The beginnings of speech. In K. Immelmann, G. W. Barlow, L. Petrinovich, & M. Main, (Eds.), *Behavioral development*, (pp. 533–561). New York: Cambridge University Press.

Thelen, E. (1986). Development of coordinated movement: implications for early human development. In M. G. Wade & H. T. A. Whiting, (Eds.). *Motor development in children: aspects of coordination and control*, (pp. 107–124). Dordrecht: Martinus Nijhoff.

Weston, J. A., Climent, G., & Girdlestone, J. (1984). The role of extracellular matrix in neural crest development: a reevaluation. In R. L. Trelstad, (Ed.), *The role of extracellular matrix in development*, (pp. 433–460). New York: Alan R. Liss.

Woolsey, T. A., Durham, D., Harris, R. M., Simons, D. J., & Valentino, K. L. (1981). Somatosensory development. In *Development of perception*, vol. 1, (pp. 259–292). New York: Academic Press.

Mechanism and Function of Cyclicity in Spontaneous Movement

Steven S. Robertson
*Department of Human Development
and Family Studies
Cornell University
Ithaca, New York*

Oscillations in biological systems are ubiquitous from the cellular to the population levels and across species (Aschoff, 1981). They vary enormously in the characteristic frequency of oscillation (milliseconds to years), the nature of the oscillation (glycolysis to mating), and the degree to which the oscillation is coupled to factors in the internal or external environment (sucking and core body temperature). Clearly, any theory of the spontaneous activity of living systems must account for these fundamental temporal patterns. Whether the oscillation is a central and defining property of the system, or merely extra biological baggage, its causes and consequences demand explanation.

Many of the oscillations in biological systems have cycle times that approximate cycles in the physical environment, which in turn reflect geologic, lunar, and solar cycles. These "circa-rhythms" (Aschoff, 1967; Halberg, 1959), and their underlying mechanisms, have been intensively studied by chronobiologists (Aschoff, 1981; Rusak & Zucker, 1975). One beneficial consequence of biological oscillations corresponding to environmental cycles seems clear: they appear to increase the organism's success in responding to predictable changes in environmental conditions such as nightfall, high tide, and winter. Not all biological oscillations, however, are linked in an obvious way to environmental cycles.

One large class of *non*-circa oscillations consists of ultradian rhythms with cycle times shorter than 24 hours. Common examples of ultradian cyclicity in the behavior of small mammals are short-term oscillations in activity, with cycle times ranging from 20 minutes to 6 hours, which are often related to foraging and food intake (Daan & Aschoff, 1981). The so-called "basic rest-activity cycle" in the human infant (Aserinsky & Kleitman, 1955), with a cycle time near 1 hour, may also be related to feeding, although in a more complicated and indirect way through its interaction with the longer sleep-wake cycle.

In immature animals, including humans, another short-term biological oscillation at the behavioral level is the cyclic fluctuation of spontaneous motor activity (comprised of general movements of the limbs, trunk, and head, and more isolated or stereotyped movements), with a cycle time of a few minutes (Corner, 1977; Hamburger, 1963; Robertson, 1985, 1987; Smotherman, Robinson & Robertson, 1988), illustrated in Figure 1. In contrast to the circa-rhythms and other ultradian oscillations in behavioral activation, cyclic motor activity (CM) in the 1−10 minute range has been studied by behavioral embryologists and psychobiologists rather than chronobiologists. CM may be a very common and robust property of the developing motor system in a variety of species (Robertson, 1985), yet it appears to be unrelated to regular temporal variations in the environment.

What is the nature of the mechanism underlying the cyclic fluctuation in spontaneous motor activity, and does CM have any psychobiological consequences? In considering these fundamental questions, I will speculate freely, subscribing to Strunk's philosophy that "it is better to be wrong than irresolute" (Strunk & White, 1979). First, however, there are some matters of definition that must be addressed.

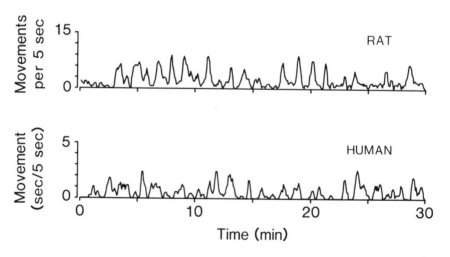

Figure 1. Time series of spontaneous motor activity. The rat fetus was observed on day 20 of gestation in a saline bath with the umbilical connection to the placenta and placental-uterine attachment intact. The time series plots the number of movements in successive 5 second intervals (Smotherman et al., 1988). The human fetus was studied at 39 weeks of gestation using strain gauges on the mother's abdomen. The time series plots the duration of movement in successive 5 second intervals (Robertson, 1987). Both series have been smoothed with a 3-term moving average filter to reduce the visual effects of high frequency variation. See Fig. 2.

DEFINITIONS

The spontaneous motor activity illustrated in Figure 1 comes and goes on a more or less regular basis. These fluctuations can be quantified by simply measuring the *duration* of motor activity in successive intervals of fixed size. When motor activity consists of relatively brief movements it may make more sense to count their *number* in successive intervals to obtain a measure of movement density as a function of time. Taking either approach, spontaneous motor activity increases and decreases repeatedly over successive intervals. It is cyclic in the sense implied by the word's etymology: the Greek *kylos* meaning circle or wheel.

On close examination, the fluctuations in the density of movement are noisy. But overall, they reveal a regularity in the envelope of change over time. Smoothing operations applied to the raw measurements highlight the envelope (Figure 2). They also show that the fluctuations in spontaneous movement, even with the more rapid variations suppressed, are not *rhythmic*. The term rhythmic implies strong regularity in the period of the cycle, as in music. Thus rhythmic variation is a special case of cyclic variation in which the cycle time is highly regulated. The relative invariance in the period of certain biological oscillations, such as circadian rhythms and normal cardiac pacemaker activity, does *not* characterize the fluctuations in spontaneous motor activity.

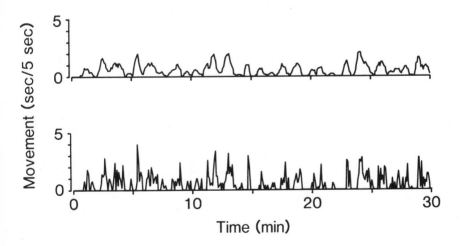

Figure 2.   The lower series is the unsmoothed data for the human fetus in Fig. 1. The upper series has been smoothed with a 5-term moving average filter.

A characteristic feature of CM, also visible in the data of Figure 1, is the continuous nature of the fluctuations in activity. CM is not, in general, a burst-pause phenomenon, in which phases of activity alternate with extended phases of complete inactivity, as in the temporal distribution of nonnutritive sucking movements in the human newborn. Burst-pause organization is a special case of the more general notion of cyclic organization, one that applies only sometimes to the fluctuations in spontaneous motor activity.

It may be that the operational definition of cyclicity in terms of bursts and pauses, or phases of activity and inactivity, can obscure the temporal organization inherent in spontaneous movement. For example, the ultrasonic visualization of human fetal movement in the first half of gestation (deVries, Visser, & Prechtl, 1982) reveals a temporal patterning in general motor activity. The periodicity has a burst-pause quality and is seen most clearly between 10 and 12 weeks, but becomes obscured after 14 weeks, being "replaced by much longer epochs of fluctuating activity." It is possible that the fluctuations retain the periodicity characteristic of the earlier burst-pause organization. As illustrated in Figure 3, the addition of a critical level of background motor activity can virtually eliminate the pauses and hence the burst-pause organization without altering the cyclic variation in general motor activity. Furthermore, the strength and frequency of the cyclic modulation may be quantitatively unchanged.

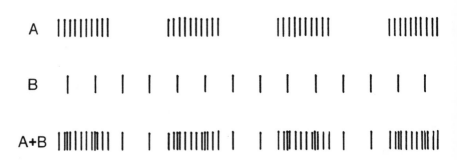

Figure 3. The effects of adding a constant level of background movement to a burst-pause pattern. The upper panel (A) shows clear burst-pause organization. The middle panel (B) represents background movements occurring at slightly less than the minimum criterion for a pause. The top two panels are superimposed in the lower panel (A+B). The result has the same cyclic fluctuation in the density of movements, but no burst-pause organization.

If the early burst-pause pattern becomes replaced by the more general phenomenon of cyclic modulation, with little or no quantitative change in basic parameters such as the frequency of the fluctuations, then a possibility of considerable theoretical interest arises. The stable cyclic organization of spontaneous motor activity observed in the human fetus after midgestation (Robertson, 1987), which persists unchanged in the newborn during active sleep (Robertson, 1987), may be continuous with the earliest burst-pause organization evident by 10 weeks (deVries et al., 1982). The demonstration of such a continuity would, in turn, guide our thinking about the neural substrate of CM in the human fetus. Furthermore, continuity in CM, while not constituting evidence of its functional significance, would provide additional motivation to discover whether it has any consequences for fetal neurobehavioral development.

The burst-pause approach to defining periodicity may also influence the quantitative estimation of one of the most basic parameters of cyclic organization, the rate or frequency of oscillation. Referring again to Figure 3, it is apparent that fluctuation in the added background noise might result in periodic pauses that meet an arbitrary duration criterion, say 10 seconds. If, however, there is an increase in total motor activity during some stages of development, then the length of the active phase (and hence the cycle time) would appear to increase as 10 sec periods of quiescence become more rare. This may explain some of the reported increase in the length of the active phase and cycle time in the spontaneous motility of the chick embryo during the middle third of incubation (Hamburger, Balaban, Oppenheim & Wenger, 1965).

The operational definition of cyclicity may therefore have a profound effect on how we address the questions of development, neural substrate, and function. In addition, defining cyclicity in a more general way rather than in terms of the special case of burst-pause organization may reveal stability rather than change in fundamental parameters such as the rate of oscillation (Robertson, 1985). This, in turn, would guide the construction of more formal theoretical models of CM as described in the next section.

MECHANISM

A satisfactory explanation of CM will have to include an understanding of the mechanism underlying its characteristic cyclic organization. Furthermore, the mechanism question will have to be addressed regardless of the functional significance (or insignificance) and evolutionary origins of CM. For example, the apparent ubiquity of CM may be unrelated to any beneficial consequences it may have. Cyclicity might, instead, be a conservative property of the developing motor system, or may itself be a necessary consequence of some more basic property of the immature motor system. However, regardless of CM's status as phenomenon or epiphenomenon, its underlying mechanism needs to be elucidated.

There are at least three different approaches that may be taken to investigate the control of CM. One is to identify the neural substrate responsible for the cyclic fluctuations in spontaneous motor activity. A second is to determine which factors in the external and internal environments influence the expression or development of CM. A third approach is to construct a formal, theoretical model of CM which accounts for its main characteristics and predicts other properties that can be tested empirically.

Neural Substrate

Evidence for the spinal origin of CM comes from a series of elegant studies of the chick embryo by Hamburger and his colleagues beginning more than 20 years ago. These studies were designed to investigate the role of sensory and supraspinal input on the motility of the chick embryo, which begins very early in incubation and is periodic from the start. Removal of the dorsal half of the lumbar spinal cord including the neural crest did not eliminate leg motility nor abolish its periodicity in embryos with entire sections of the thoracic cord removed (Hamburger, Wenger, & Oppenheim, 1966). The neurogenic nature of spontaneous movements in the chick embryo was demonstrated by the simultaneous recording of multiunit burst discharges in the ventral portion of the spinal cord during overt movements (Provine & Rogers, 1977; Ripley & Provine, 1972).

Thus CM in the chick embryo appears to be generated in the spinal cord without afferent input or input from the brain. However, by mid-incubation an early and chronic gap in the cervical spinal cord results in motility cycles that have shorter active phases and longer inactive phases, with no change in the total number of movements, suggesting a role of supraspinal structures in the temporal patterning of spinal motor output (Oppenheim, 1975). Similar effects were seen at a slightly younger age in embryos with a gap in the thoracic portion of the spinal cord, demonstrating that input from other parts of the cord as well as from the brain serve to modulate CM.

Qualitative descriptions of the movements of anencephalic fetuses early in gestation suggest that human CM may also be generated in the cord and modulated by supraspinal structures (Visser, Laurini, deVries, Bekedam, & Prechtl, 1985). The normal burst-pause characteristic of spontaneous fetal movement observed during the first trimester of gestation using ultrasound techniques (deVries, et al., 1982) appears exaggerated in anencephalic fetuses and persists during subsequent weeks when the simple burst-pause quality of motility disappears in the normal fetus (Visser et al, 1985). Taken together, these observations suggest the burst-pause organization might originate in the spinal cord and interact with descending input from supraspinal structures by the end of the first trimester of gestation. The relevance of these observations to speculation about the neural substrate of human fetal and newborn CM (Robertson, 1985, 1987) depends in part on whether a link can be found between the early burst-pause characteristic of spontaneous fetal movement and the cyclic property of fluctuations in motor activity later in gestation.

The development of human CM during the second half of gestation and into the early postnatal period seems to be consistent with the view that the cyclic variation in spontaneous motor activity is spinal in origin, but is influenced by the brain. One of the most striking features of fetal CM is the quantitative stability in the basic parameters describing its cyclic organization during the third trimester of gestation. This is a period when other aspects of neurobehavioral organization controlled by supraspinal structures (e.g., sleep-wake state organization) are undergoing rapid developmental change. After birth, CM in active sleep is nearly identical to fetal CM, but differs consistently from CM in the non-sleep states (Robertson, 1987). The nature of the differences (e.g., decreased strength and regularity in active sleep) suggests that spinal circuits controlling CM may be influenced by the strong, phasic, descending input from the brain stem which occurs during active sleep (Vertes, 1984). However, the *rate* of oscillation is the least affected of all the parameters. This raises the possibility that the mechanism responsible for the cyclic temporal organization of motility is different than the circuits generating the motor output. That is, an oscillatory mechanism or mechanisms may produce CM by modulating the ongoing level of spontaneous motor activity. The hypothesis that the control of the cyclicity and level of motor activity are independent is supported by the fact that the parameters of CM do not differ among the nonsleep states (from drowsy to crying) in spite of enormous differences in the *amount* of movement.

A recent study suggests that the fetal rat may be a useful animal model with which to explore the neural substrate of CM (Smotherman, et al., 1988). In that study, methods for the direct observation of fetal rat behavior (Smotherman, Richards, & Robinson, 1984) were combined with analytic techniques for detecting and quantifying cyclicity in spontaneous motor activity (Robertson, 1985). The results revealed cyclic organization in 17 of 19 fetuses studied. Quantitative differences were found between rat and human fetal CM, but they appear to be minor. The results therefore provide the behavioral justification for subsequent experiments aimed at determining the neural substrate of CM in the rat. Spontaneous complex discharges in explants of fetal mouse and rat spinal cord and medulla have been observed to exhibit a periodicity of a few minutes (Corner & Crain, 1972). Furthermore, the sensitivity of these preparations to electrical stimulation was also found to fluctuate, even in cultures which did not exhibit spontaneous discharges, suggesting the periodicity might be due to cyclic variation in some threshold. Three questions of particular importance to address in subsequent neurobehavioral studies of the rat fetus, therefore, will be (a) whether the cyclicity in spontaneous motor activity is spinal in origin, (b) to what extent supraspinal structures regulate or modulate the cyclicity, and (c) whether the control of the cyclicity and level of activity are separate.

Factors which Influence CM

A second approach to investigating the control of cyclicity in spontaneous movement is primarily empirical in nature. It consists of accumulating evidence about which factors in the external and internal environments influence the expression or development of CM. Although the initial motivation for these investigations is relatively atheoretical, the results may provide a useful empirical base from which to generate specific hypotheses about the nature of the mechanism controlling CM. In addition, the results will put real constraints on more abstract or formal models of CM.

Very little is known about the factors that influence CM. In the human, fetal CM is disrupted by maternal diabetes (Robertson & Dierker, 1986). At the beginning of the third trimester of gestation, the rate of oscillation in the CM of fetuses of insulin dependent diabetic mothers is slower than in normal fetuses. Subsequent increases in the rate of CM to normal values suggests the initial differences might reflect a slight developmental delay. The effects of maternal diabetes on fetal CM are more pronounced when the mother's blood glucose levels during the third trimester are less well controlled. Thus, the mechanism controlling fetal CM in the third trimester appears to be sensitive to some aspect of the prenatal environment altered by maternal hyperglycemia, or factors that covary with maternal blood glucose levels.

A second set of effects, also linked to maternal hyperglycemia, emerges around 36 weeks of gestation. Since this is a time when fetal state organization is maturing rapidly (Nijhuis, Prechtl, Martin, & Bots, 1982) and may be sensitive to disruption, these transient effects of maternal diabetes on fetal CM may be mediated by atypical state organization and the resulting alterations in the pattern of supraspinal input to the mechanism controlling CM.

A major unanswered question is whether the sensitivity of CM to maternal diabetes is a short-term, physiologic response to changes in the metabolic environment, or a reflection of subtle alterations in neural organization occurring early in the first trimester. The latter possibility must be seriously considered, since (a) the congenital malformations, including those of the CNS, which are more common in infants of diabetic mothers, occur during the first 6 weeks of gestation (Mills, Baker, & Goldman, 1979), and (b) the reduction in morbidity due to aggressive management of diabetes in pregnancy after the first trimester has not been matched by similar reductions in the incidence of malformations (Ballard, Holroyde, Tsang, Chan, Sutherland, & Knowles, 1984). The normalization of CM in fetuses of diabetic mothers by the end of gestation, which persists after birth, suggests that the mechanism controlling CM ultimately recovers and remains buffered from the effects of maternal diabetes (Robertson, 1988).

Model of CM

A third approach to understanding the control of CM is to build a general model that accounts for its main characteristics (spontaneous and sustained oscillations) and predicts other properties that can be tested empirically. As in other attempts to construct general models of biological oscillations (e.g., Pavlidis, 1973; Pittendrigh & Bruce, 1957; Winfree, 1980), some of the questions to address are: (a) Can the control of CM be adequately described by a simple clock model with phase as the only variable, or is a second variable such as amplitude required? If so, does the mechanism have a preferred amplitude (attracting cycle)? (b) Is there a single source of oscillation, or are multiple oscillators implicated? (c) If multiple oscillators are implicated, are they relatively independent or coupled? Can some of the noisy character of human CM be explained as incoherence among units in a multioscillator system? (d) Is the mechanism controlling CM capable of entrainment with an external stimulus?

A general model would provide a theoretical framework within which to investigate the properties of CM (e.g., entrainment). More important, it might provide unified explanations of empirical observations concerning the development, control, and function of CM. For example, some of the developmental changes in fetal CM early in the third trimester, such as increased strength (Robertson, 1985), might be explained as increased coupling among elements in a multioscillator system. The disruption of the rate of oscillation, more than its strength, in fetuses of diabetic mothers (Robertson & Dierker, 1986) might be explained in terms of differential phase and amplitude sensitivities of the model.

A general model such as one that included multiple coupled oscillators instead of a single source of oscillation would guide experimental attempts to define the neural substrate of CM. In turn, empirical findings about the neural substrate of CM might constitute critical tests of the general model. Finally, if the model suggested the possibility of entrainment (e.g., phase sensitivity) by an external stimulus, there would be additional reason to investigate the role of postnatal CM in infant-environment interactions in studies of its possible psychobiological functions. Quantitative experimental data on phase sensitivity might even suggest which natural stimuli (social or otherwise) might be effective.

A very different approach to modeling temporal patterns in motor activity (not specifically CM) has been proposed by Lehmann (1976). At the core of this approach is the assumption that fluctuations in activity can be represented by a binary process—a series of alternating periods of activity and inactivity, perhaps with separate controls. There are numerous reasons why this approach is not appropriate for CM. A major and sufficient reason is that CM is not a burst-pause phenomenon. At the behavioral level (see Figure 1) there is no compelling reason to view the fluctuations in spontaneous motility as the result of a single binary process. Rather, the empirical evidence obtained from both the human (Robertson, 1985) and rat fetus (Smotherman et al., 1988), and other species (Corner, 1977), indicates that CM consists of continuous fluctuations in motor activity superimposed on a background which may or may not be silent. It is these fluctuations which must be accounted for by a general model.

In constructing a model it will be important to distinguish between the quantities that can be observed in experiments and the variables of the underlying mechanism (e.g. Pittendrigh & Bruce, 1957), since the connection between the two can be complex. For CM, frequency (rate) and strength are two observable properties that have logical, empirical, and intuitive appeal. Logically, frequency is an important variable because it is related to phase (as the first time derivative), which is perhaps the most central and defining feature of any cyclic phenomenon. Similarly, the strength of CM is a logical first choice as a measure of the amplitude of the underlying oscillation, if this turns out to be an important variable in the model. Empirically, frequency and strength have proven to be useful descriptors of fetal and newborn CM since both vary and they appear to be statistically independent. Intuitively, the rate and strength of an oscillation capture its most salient properties.

A reasonable assumption to make at the beginning is that the basic process underlying the oscillations in motor activity is not deterministic but stochastic. That is, there is no reason to assume at the outset that the output of the underlying process is a unique, single-valued function of time or past output. More realistically, based on the quantitative behavioral data that are available (e.g., Robertson, 1985; Smotherman, et al., 1988) and the general nature of biological systems, there is likely to be a strong probabilistic component to the process underlying CM. Thus some inherent variability in the fundamental parameters of the process would be expected. This would lead to variability in the observable properties of CM even under ideal conditions of close correspondence (direct and noiseless) between the observable properties and underlying parameters.

As others (e.g., Pavlidis, 1971) have pointed out, the characteristics of the mechanism underlying a biological oscillation that distinguish it from other plausible mechanisms can often be observed best in unnatural circumstances. Presumably any model worth considering will account for the usual, undisturbed behavior of the system. The task is how to select among them. One approach is to observe the system's response to a perturbation. In the study of biological oscillations, such "resetting" experiments have often been used to gain considerable insight into the nature of the underlying mechanism (Winfree, 1980).

Resetting experiments on CM might therefore be devised to focus on the frequency and strength of the fluctuations in spontaneous motility, and how they are affected by a pulse-like stimulus that activates the motor system. The absence of any effects on the strength of CM would raise the possibility that the underlying mechanism behaves as a single, simple clock which can be completely specified by its phase, with no need to consider a second variable such as amplitude. These results would also be consistent with a mechanism having variable phase and amplitude but with amplitude strongly regulated, that is, an oscillator which returns very promptly to its original amplitude (an attracting cycle) following a perturbation. A transient change in amplitude after the pulse would implicate a 2-variable model with an attracting cycle. A persistent change in strength would raise the possibility that there are two or more oscillators whose phases are dispersed by the perturbing pulse, resulting in a decrease in their aggregate amplitude.

In view of the evidence indicating that many other biological oscillations are controlled by two or more oscillators (Aschoff, 1981; Pavlidis, 1973; Winfree, 1980), a multioscillator model might also be considered for CM. The data obtained from the chick embryo demonstrate that separate sections of the spinal cord are capable of generating CM, although propriospinal influences are apparent (Oppenheim, 1975). It is characteristic of even weakly coupled nonlinear oscillators to become synchronized

(Oatley & Goodwin, 1971; Winfree, 1980). The double peak structure of some human fetal movement spectra (Robertson, Dierker, Sorokin & Rosen, 1982) is consistent with uncoupling in a dual oscillator system (or subpopulations in a multioscillator system).

FUNCTION

Do the cyclic fluctuations in spontaneous motor activity have any functional significance? Or is CM entirely without consequence? As so often happens, there are no data on which to base an empirical answer to this important question. There are, however, some bits and pieces of information from neurobehavioral studies in other areas, as well as some more general theoretical positions, which might support speculation about the possible beneficial consequences of CM—its functions in the broadest sense of the term (Hinde, 1975).

First, however, it is important to acknowledge that the apparent ubiquity of CM does not constitute evidence of its functional significance, although it certainly leaves open that possibility. Oscillation may be a nearly unavoidable property of complex systems with numerous interacting elements subjected to physical, biochemical, or other constraints. Or it may be a highly conservative property of the motor system in its early stages of development. Nevertheless, the biological inevitability of oscillation does not tell us whether it does or does not have any utility.

We can, and should, consider the possible consequences of CM separately from the question of its evolutionary origins. The neural mechanism responsible for CM may have evolved or persisted for reasons quite unrelated to any utility it might currently have (Dumont & Robertson, 1986; Jamieson, 1986). In fact, the current utility of CM—if it has any—may be entirely opportunistic, in spite of our rationalist tendency to believe otherwise (Dahlbom, 1985). And even if CM has persisted because of its advantages, we should not be tempted to adopt a whiggish view of its evolution, a process which is more like tinkering than engineering (Jacob, 1977; Partridge, 1982).

Although the distinction between function and evolution has not always been respected, numerous possible advantages or beneficial consequences of biological oscillations have been proposed. Rapp (1987) discusses many of them: oscillation can provide a means for coordinating or segregating biological processes in time and space. Intrinsic oscillation also can provide a basis for predicting repetitive external events. Furthermore, the energy efficiency of some biochemical processes may be optimal when they oscillate, and there is ample evidence for the utility of frequency modulation for encoding information, as in the nervous system.

As suggested elsewhere (Robertson, 1987) and discussed more fully below, it is the capacity of an oscillatory system to segregate beneficial but incompatible processes in time which may be a significant advantage of cyclic motor activation during early development. The segregation of incompatible processes has been considered a functional advantage in other oscillatory systems as well (Oatley & Goodwin, 1971). In general terms, Winfree (1980) argues that there appears to be "no virtue in perfect stationarity per se." Rather, fluctuation may provide a way to accommodate incompatible processes that cannot be separated in space. Moore-Ede and Sulzman (1981) also argue that periodic fluctuations of the internal environment may permit the use of the same cellular machinery at different times for processes that require different biochemical conditions.

There are widespread effects of neural and neuromuscular activity during development, including the regulation of central and neuromuscular synapses (Greenough, 1986; Harris, 1981; Oppenheim, 1981; Purves & Lichtman, 1980). There is also some evidence that periodic activity may be more effective than constant activity at the same average level (Thompson, 1983). Spontaneous activation of the immature motor system may therefore serve an important function by insuring an adequate level or pattern of neural and neuromuscular activity during its early development. Continuous high levels of activity, while in the short run being most effective in inducing the cellular processes that underlie the changes in receptor distribution, synaptic strength, and other properties, might deplete necessary substrates or reduce crucial ionic gradients. The regular alternation of periods of relative increased and decreased activity, manifested at the behavioral level by CM, could provide a means of realizing the benefits of suprathreshold activity and quiescence by segregating them in time.

Even if continuous high levels of activity are possible, the threshold for synaptic modification or other changes may increase as a function of the recent time average of the activity (Bear, Cooper, & Ebner, 1987). In that case, cyclic activation would provide a way to maintain the average level of activity, and hence the threshold for synaptic modification, at a relatively constant level below peak activity levels. Cyclic activation would result in periodic surges that exceed the modification threshold while the threshold, by virtue of the periods of quiescence, would remain stable.

In either case, cyclic activation would balance the benefits of activity and quiescence. This is not to say that cyclic activation is the only way to strike such a balance, nor that it is necessarily the best way. The point is simply that the oscillatory processes underlying CM may have beneficial consequences for the developing neuromotor system.

In this context, it may be possible to understand better some of the individual differences in the rate of cyclic motor activation observed within a single species (e.g., Robertson, 1985; Smotherman et al., 1988). Within relatively wide limits, the precise rate at which motor activity oscillates may not be important. Even though the frequency of oscillation is likely to remain a key parameter in any formal model of the mechanism underlying CM, variation in frequency will be functionally inconsequential so long as the periods of relative activity and inactivity remain within the limits required to realize their specific benefits.

The oscillation in neural and neuromuscular activity generating fetal CM may, therefore, have important consequences, quite independent of its evolutionary origins. It will be a separate problem to determine whether, and to what extent, any demonstrated benefits of cyclic motor activation have played a role in the ubiquity and persistence of CM. As Gould and Lewontin (1979) point out, "male tyrannosaurs may have used their diminutive front legs to titillate female partners, but this will not explain *why* they got so small."

In the human, however, and perhaps other species, a different challenge confronts any functional explanation of CM: the persistence of cyclic organization in spontaneous motor activity after birth (Robertson, 1987). In view of other evidence for the continuity of neural and behavioral organization across birth in the human (Prechtl, 1984), post-natal CM may be nothing more than the persistence of fetal CM. From a functional point of view, the benefits of fetal CM—if any—might also be expected to be relevant after birth, at least for awhile. However, it is reasonable to consider that postnatal CM may have beneficial consequences quite un-related to its prenatal functions, especially if one rejects a strict adaptationist approach to the functional analysis of behavior.

After birth, newborn behavior begins to play a crucial role in regulating interactions with the environment. For example, fetal behavior does not appear to directly influence the supply of fuels and other nutrients. Instead, continuous placental transfer fluctuates in response to maternal meals and metabolism. However, newborn behavior plays a key role in regulating nutrient intake. It is partly the periodic changes in newborn behavior that elicit intermittent oral feedings from the mother.

Cyclic motor activity may undergo a similar functional metamorphosis after birth. In particular, CM may regulate the infant's interaction with its physical and social environment. A functional analysis in terms of the temporal segregation of incompatible processes might serve as a useful starting point for postnatal CM, just as it may provide insight into the function of fetal CM (Polya, 1973). For example, relative motor quiescence during awake periods might permit or facilitate attention to visual or auditory information in the environment, while increased motor activity might elicit responses from adult caregivers or trigger shifts in the infant's focus of attention in an unchanging stimulus environment. Cyclic fluctuations in motor activity therefore might balance the benefits of action and attention.

As before, there is no reason to think that CM, even if it has beneficial consequences on infant-environment interaction, is the primary or best source of regulation. It might, however, serve as one relatively automatic source of regulation in the first few weeks after birth before the increase in more goal-directed, intentional behavior (Hopkins & Prechtl, 1984; Wolff, 1984).

These speculations about the functional consequences of postnatal CM in regulating interaction with the environment also suggest a more parsimonious view of newborn state organization. Non-crying awake time has traditionally been thought to consist of two separate and distinct states: quiet and active, with quiet awake states characterized by apparently attentive visual behaviors such as fixation and scanning (e.g., Prechtl, 1974). Quiet awakeness is typically of short duration, however, and may simply correspond to the relatively inactive phase of CM during which sustained attention to the environment is increased. Thus it may be more accurate to think of awake time as a single state during which behavioral activation fluctuates with a cycle time of a few minutes. The quantitative similarity in the parameters of CM during awake, fussy, and crying periods (Robertson, 1987) raises the possibility that all non-sleep states, from quiet awake to crying, should be considered a single state on a continuum of increasing behavioral activation, the level of which is modulated by the mechanism responsible for CM.

CONCLUSION

A better understanding of cyclicity in spontaneous movement will come from trying to answer questions about (a) its developmental origin and fate, (b) the nature of the mechanism responsible for the characteristic cyclicity, (c) the psychobiological consequences of cyclic motor activation, and (d) the evolutionary origins of CM. In this essay I have focused attention on two of these fundamental questions, mechanism and function, but the interrelatedness of them all is difficult to miss. Ultimately the goal is to achieve an integrated rather than piecemeal knowledge of this biological oscillation, which will require more than collecting empirical observations relevant to the four questions. It will require theory construction. I have particularly high hopes for mathematical models and the way "number holds sway above the flux" (Russell, 1951), and for the value of cracks, cavities, and singularities in the predictions of those models. Sherlock Holmes apparently claimed that "singularity is almost invariably a clue" (Winfree, 1980). We shall see.

Acknowledgements

The work on human cyclic motility has been supported in part by NIH grants HD11089, RR00210, and HD18265, with the expert assistance of the staff of the Perinatal Clinical Research Center at Cleveland Metropolitan General Hospital and S. Carrel. I thank M. Robertson, as usual, for her comments on the manuscript.

References

Aschoff, J. (1967). Adaptive cycles: Their significance for defining environmental hazards. *International Journal of Biometeorology, 11*, 255–278.

Aschoff, J. (Ed.). (1981). *Handbook of Behavioral Neurobiology, Vol. 4: Biological Rhythms.* New York: Plenum.

Aserinsky, E., & Kleitman, N. (1955). A motility cycle in sleeping infants as manifested by ocular and gross bodily activity. *Journal of Applied Physiology, 8*, 11–18.

Ballard, J. L., Holroyde, J., Tsang, R.C., Chan, G., Sutherland, J.M., & Knowles, H. C. (1984). High malformation rates and decreased mortality in infants of diabetic mothers managed after the first trimester of pregnancy (1956–1978). *American Journal of Obstetrics and Gynecology, 148*, 1111– 1118.

Bear, M. F., Cooper, L. N., & Ebner, F. F. (1987). A physiological basis for a theory of synapse modification. *Science, 237*, 42–48.

Corner, M. A. (1977). Sleep and the beginnings of behavior in the animal kingdom—studies of ultradian motility cycles in early life. *Progress in Neurobiology., 8*, 279–295.

Corner, M. A., & Crain, S. M. (1972). Patterns of spontaneous bioelectric activity during maturation in culture of fetal rodent medulla and spinal cord tissues. *Journal of Neurobiology, 3*, 25–45.

Daan, S., & Aschoff, J. (1981). Short-term rhythms in activity. In J. Aschoff (Ed.), *Handbook of Behavioral Neurobiology, Vol. 4: Biological Rhythms* (pp. 491–498). New York: Plenum.

Dahlbom, B. (1985). Dennett on cognitive ethology: a broader view. *The Behavioral and Brain Sciences, 8*: 760–762.

deVries, J. I. P., Visser, G. H. A., & Prechtl, H. F. R. (1982). The emergence of fetal behaviour. I. Qualitative aspects. *Early Human Development, 7*, 301–322.

Dumont, J. P. C., & Robertson, R. M. (1986). Neuronal circuits: an evolutionary perspective. *Science, 233*, 849–853.

Gould, S. J., & Lewontin, R. C. (1979). The spandrels of San Marco and the Panglossian paradigm: a critique of the adaptationist programme. *Proceedings of the Royal Society of London, B205*, 581–598.

Greenough, W. T. (1986). What's special about development? Thoughts on the bases of experience-sensitive synaptic plasticity. In W. T. Greenough & J. M. Juraska (Eds.), *Developmental Neuropsychobiology* (pp. 387–407). New York: Academic Press.

Halberg, F. (1959). Physiologic 24-hour periodicity: General and procedural considerations with reference to the adrenal cycle. *Zeitschrift fur Vitamin-, Hormon- und Fermentforschung, 10*, 225–296.

Hamburger, V. (1963). Some aspects of the embryology of behavior. *Quarterly Review of Biology, 38*, 342–365.

Hamburger, V., Balaban, M., Oppenheim, R., & Wenger, E. (1965). Periodic motility of normal and spinal chick embryos between 8 and 17 days of incubation. *Journal of Experimental Zoology, 159*, 1–14.

Hamburger, V., Wenger, E., & Oppenheim, R. (1966). Motility in the chick embryo in the absence of sensory input. *Journal of Experimental Zoology, 162*, 133–160.

Harris, W. A. (1981). Neural activity and development. *Annual Review of Physiology, 43*, 689–710.

Hinde, R. A. (1975). The concept of function. In G. Baerends, C. Beer, and A. Manning (Eds.), *Function and Evolution in Behaviour (pp. 3–15)*. Oxford: Clarendon Press.

Hopkins, B., & Prechtl, H. F. R. (1984). A qualitative approach to the development of movements during early infancy. In H. F. R. Prechtl (Ed.), *Continuity of Neural Functions From Prenatal to Postnatal Life* (Clinics in Developmental Medicine No. 94) (pp. 179–197) Philadelphia: Lippincott.

Jacob, F. (1977). Evolution and tinkering. *Science, 196*, 1161–1166.

Jamieson, I. G. (1986). The functional approach to behavior: is it useful? *American Naturalist, 127*, 195–208.

Lehmann, U. (1976). Stochastic principles in the temporal control of activity behaviour. *International Journal of Chronobiology, 4*, 223–266.

Mills, J. L., Baker, L., & Goldman, A. S. (1979). Malformations in infants of diabetic mothers occur before the seventh gestational week. *Diabetes, 28*, 292–293.

Moore-Ede, M. C., & Sulzman, F. M. (1981). Internal temporal order. In J. Aschoff (Ed.), *Handbook of Behavioral Neurobiology, Vol. 4: Biological Rhythms* (pp. 215–241). New York: Plenum.

Nijhuis, J. G., Prechtl, H. F. R.., Martin, C. B., & Bots, R. S. G. M. (1982). Are there behavioral states in the human fetus? *Early Human Development, 6*, 177–195.

Oatley, K., & Goodwin, B. C. (1971). The explanation and investigation of biological rhythms. In W. P. Colquhoun (Ed.), *Biological Rhythms and Human Performance* (pp. 1–38). London: Academic Press.

Oppenheim, R. W. (1975). The role of supraspinal input in embryonic motility: A reexamination in the chick. *Journal of Comparative Neurology, 160*, 37–50.

Oppenheim, R. W. (1981). Neuronal cell death and some related regressive phenomena during neurogenesis: a selective historical review and progress report. In W. M. Cowan (Ed.), *Studies in Developmental Neurobiology: Essays in Honor of Viktor Hamburger* (pp. 74–133). New York: Oxford University Press.

Partridge, L. D. (1982). The good enough calculi of evolving control systems: evolution is not engineering. *American Journal of Physiology, 242*, R173–R177.

Pavlidis, T. (1971). Populations of biochemical oscillators as circadian clocks. *Journal of Theoretical Biology, 33*, 319–338.

Pavlidis, T. (1973). *Biological Oscillators: Their Mathematical Analysis*. New York: Academic Press.

Pittendrigh, C. S., & Bruce, V. (1957). An oscillator model for biological clocks. In D. Rudnick (Ed.), *Rhythmic and Synthetic Processes in Growth* (pp. 75–109). New Jersey: Princeton University Press.

Polya, G. (1973). *How to Solve It* (2nd ed.). Princeton: Princeton University Press.

Prechtl, H. F. R. (1974). The behavioral states of the newborn infant. *Brain Research, 76,* 185–212.

Prechtl, H. F. R. (1984). Continuity and change in early neural development. In H. F. R. Prechtl (Ed.), *Continuity of Neural Functions From Prenatal to Postnatal Life.* (Clinics in Developmental Medicine No. 94) (pp. 1–15). Philadelphia: Lippincott.

Provine, R. R., & Rogers, L. (1977). Development of spinal cord bioelectric activity in spinal chick embryos and its behavioral implications. *Journal of Neurobiology, 8,* 217–228.

Purves, D., & Lichtman, J. W. (1980). Elimination of synapses in the developing nervous system. *Science, 210,* 153–157.

Rapp, P. E. (1987). Why are so many biological systems periodic? *Progress in Neurobiology, 29,* 261–273.

Ripley, K. L., & Provine, R. R. (1972). Neural correlates of embryonic motility in the chick. *Brain Research, 46,* 127–134.

Robertson, S. S. (1985). Cyclic motor activity in the human fetus after midgestation. *Developmental Psychobiology, 18,* 411–419.

Robertson, S. S. (1987). Human cyclic motility: Fetal-newborn continuities and newborn state differences. *Developmental Psychobiology, 20,* 425–442.

Robertson, S. S. (1988). Infants of diabetic mothers: Late normalization of fetal cyclic motility persists after birth. *Developmental Psychobiology, 21,* 477–490.

Robertson, S. S., & Dierker, L. J. (1986). The development of cyclic motility in fetuses of diabetic mothers. *Developmental Psychobiology, 19,* 223–234.

Robertson, S. S., Dierker, L. J., Sorokin, Y., & Rosen, M. G. (1982). Human fetal movement: spontaneous oscillations near one cycle per minute. *Science, 218,* 1327–1330.

Rusak, B., & Zucker, I. (1975). Biological rhythms and animal behavior. *Annual Review of Psychology, 26,* 137–171.

Russell, B. (1951). *The Autobiography of Bertrand Russell, 1972–1914.* Boston: Little, Brown & Co.

Smotherman, W. P., Richards, L. S., & Robinson, S. R. (1984) Techniques for observing fetal behavior in utero: A comparison of chemomyelotomy and spinal transection. *Developmental Psychobiology, 17,* 661–674.

Smotherman, W. P., Robinson, S. R., & Robertson, S. S. (1988). Cyclic motor activity in the rat fetus. *Journal of Comparative Psychology, 102,* 78–82.

Strunk, W., Jr., & White, E. B. (1979). *The Elements of Style* (3rd ed.). New York: Macmillan Co.

Thompson, W. (1983). Synapse elimination in neonatal rat muscle is sensitive to pattern of muscle use. *Nature, 302,* 614–616.

Visser, G. H. A., Laurini, R. N., deVries, J. I. P., Bekedam, D. J., & Prechtl, H. F. R. (1985). Abnormal motor behaviour in anencephalic fetuses. *Early Human Development, 12,* 173–182.

Winfree, A. T. (1980). *The Geometry of Biological Time.* New York: Springer-Verlag.

Wolff. P. H. (1984). Discontinuous changes in human wakefulness around the end of the second month of life: a developmental perspective. In H. F. R. Prechtl (Ed.), *Continuity of Neural Functions From Prenatal to Postnatal Life* (Clinics in Developmental Medicine No. 94) (pp. 144–158). Philadelphia: Lippincott.

Chance and Chunks in the Ontogeny of Fetal Behavior

Scott R. Robinson and William P. Smotherman
Laboratory for Psychobiological Research *Department of Psychology*
Department of Zoology *State University of New York*
Oregon State University *Binghamton, New York*
Corvallis, Oregon

In the course of communicating the findings of our fetal research to scientific and lay audiences alike, the subject that invariably elicits the most comment is the image of a living fetus. Relationships and patterns of significance may pique the intellect, but a visual image evokes wonder. The advent of noninvasive technology that permits visualization of human fetuses and improvements in surgical and experimental procedures for viewing nonhuman fetuses has created unprecedented access for observing fetuses *in vivo*. It is the thesis of this essay that, in addition to inspiring awe and curiosity, much stands to be learned from the observational study of fetal behavior.

Early observations by behavioral embryologists (e.g., Coghill, 1929; Windle, 1944) engendered much discussion of general principles in the process of prenatal behavioral development. But the conceptual dichotomies created by these early workers, such as the distinction between integration and differentiation in behavioral development, proved to be simplistic and intellectually sterile. Observational study of fetuses was virtually nonexistent between 1940 and 1970.

Overlapping this period of stasis was the discovery of DNA, the mechanisms regulating embryological development, the existence of teratogens, the diversity and complexity of neurochemistry, the processes of maternal-fetal physiology, and a host of other phenomena fundamental to fetal development. Perhaps because these new fields offered such promise, and perhaps because earlier workers had claimed to have seen all there was to see in the behavior of fetuses, the observation of fetal behavior remained an historical curiosity until the widespread use of automatic recording devices (see Robertson, this volume) and ultrasonographic imaging (see Birnholz, this volume). As the chapters in this volume attest, the observational study of prenatal behavior is once again a thriving, rapidly growing field.

LEVELS OF BEHAVIORAL DESCRIPTION

'Behavior' is a shorthand word that is used to refer to overt expressions of the functioning of a complex system of neurons and muscles. Some investigators have argued that inferences drawn from observation of behavior are inadequate as a basis for firm conclusions about the presence or absence of underlying neural or motor organization. What is needed, they claim, is a more reductionist investigation of organization at the neurophysiological level. This emphasis is proper if one is primarily interested in neural mechanisms. And it is certainly true that neuroethological approaches have and will continue to offer valuable perspectives on problems of behavioral control. But emphasizing neurophysiological questions and methods in explicit preference to observation of overt behavior obscures the broad objective of understanding the development and organization of behavior.

There is a more basic difficulty with abandoning behavioral study for the allure of neurophysiological objectivity. The obverse face of this question may be referred to as the "degrees of freedom problem." Behavior consists, at the neurophysiological level of description, of stimulation or inhibition of activity in individual motor units. The human body, to select a representative animal at nonrandom, comprises nearly 800 muscles distributed among over 100 flexible joints. The description of a behavioral event at the level of muscles and joints therefore could require specification of an expression consisting of roughly 10^3 terms, each of which could vary continuously within a range of values and change from moment to moment. It was recognition of the problem of degrees of freedom that led Weiss (1941) and others (e.g., Dawkins, 1976; Kugler et al., 1982; Fentress, 1983) to argue that the neuromotor system must be organized in a hierarchy of levels. Since Weiss presented his six-level scheme of neural organization many neural structures that function at hierarchical levels above that of the individual motor unit have been identified. But high-level neural correlates typically have been discovered not through naive neurological exploration, but confirmed after their existence was inferred from overt behavioral data.

The reverse face of the same problem is the technology of measurement. Ideally, a pattern of motor behavior could be uniquely specified by measuring the degree of muscle contraction in all motor units involved in the pattern. But even if a limited pattern of behavior (one involving only a handful of motor units) formed the focus of study, the current technical reality of recording simultaneously from multiple muscles is that the overall form of a behavioral event cannot be reconstructed from neurophysiological data. The degree of muscle contraction must be inferred from the strength of the EMG signal, which also varies as a function of electrode placement, characteristics of individual muscles, physical/mechanical context, etc. Quantitatively relating many different EMG signals therefore is too imprecise to permit specification of, say, the relative position of two limbs during their trajectory through space. The study of behavior will continue to be as important to the understanding of neurobiology as the study of the nervous system is to the understanding of behavior.

THE BASIS OF BEHAVIORAL DEVELOPMENT

Because behavior does not have a physical existence separate from neurons and muscles, it is possible that behavioral development can be explained solely by reference to cellular and tissue-level events in the neuromotor system. One can construct a functioning machine without any understanding of its functions, for example, if provided with a sufficiently detailed blueprint for attaching nuts, bolts, cams, cogs, etc. By this view, behavioral development is merely a visible manifestation of an architectural plan that is configured in neural and muscular maturation (see Smotherman & Robinson, this volume).

If, however, functioning of the neuromotor system as a whole plays any role in directing the course of development of the system, and therefore of behavior, then adequate developmental explanations must entail reference to higher levels of organization than cell-to-cell interaction (see Hofer, this volume). When function is involved in determining the development of structure, the system may be said to exhibit properties of self-organization.

The degree to which behavior exhibits self-organization during early development remains an open question. If early behavioral patterning merely reflects intrinsic organizational events within the nervous system, then descriptions of development at a behavioral level ultimately may be unnecessary. If, on the other hand, behavior exhibits self-organization during ontogeny, analysis at the behavioral level is mandatory. It is reference to the involvement of such higher levels of organization that we intend when we advocate observational analysis.

The observational study of behavioral development need not consist of qualitative behavioral commentary, such as was characteristic during the heyday of behavioral embryology (1920–1940). Rather, behavioral analysis has come to be considerably more sophisticated. Quantitative techniques borrowed from theoretical mathematics, cybernetics, physics, economics, linguistics and many other disciplines have had a profound impact in certain areas of psychology, ethology and behavioral ecology (Colgan, 1978; Sackett, 1978; Martin & Bateson, 1986). The advantage presented by these analytic techniques is that they apply specific organizational models to the complexity of behavioral output. Sometimes these approaches confirm subjective impressions of behavioral organization that is not perceptible to an observer and is not obtainable from measurement of low-level elements of the neuromotor system. The sections that follow briefly introduce how some of these observational approaches have been applied to the study of behavior before birth and, further, how they can yield fresh insights into the self-organization of behavior during early development.

PRENATAL DEVELOPMENT OF MOTOR COORDINATION

Behavioral scientists who are accustomed to working with mature subjects may tend to assume that motor behavior must involve some degree of coordination. However, subjective notions of random motility in the fetus call this assumption into question. Most of the early students of fetal behavior, and many investigators since, concluded that fetal behavior was lacking in coordination. But coordination is an inherently quantitative concept, encompassing synchronized motor activity at levels ranging from contraction of fibers within a muscle to finely tuned movements involving the entire body, that requires quantitative techniques for its characterization and explication.

When examining behavioral events that are not perfectly coordinated—a situation that applies especially to the prenatal development of behavior—it is necessary to have a standard to which observed performances can be compared. One strategy for providing a suitable standard is to compare the frequencies or rates of different behavioral performances within the same individual. This method has been effectively used by Provine (1980) in characterizing the development of interlimb coordination in chick embryos (*Gallus domesticus*). Chick embryos ranging in age from 7–19 days of incubation were observed through a small opening in the egg and individual movements of left and right wings and legs scored as independent movement events. Because the timing of each movement was preserved, it was possible to calculate the percentage of time that two limbs moved concurrently. From day 7 until about day 14, movements involving a wing and the ipsilateral leg occurred about as often as movements comprising right and left wings. After this time, wing-wing movements increased sharply in frequency as wing-leg synchrony diminished. This quantitative demonstration of emergent coordination between wings thus depends upon explicit comparison to a standard presumed to lack coordination (wing-leg synchrony).

The issue of interlimb coordination in mammalian fetuses has been addressed by Bekoff and Lau (1980) in a study of rats (*Rattus norvegicus*) on embryonic day 20, the penultimate day of gestation. Observation consisted of filming fetuses that had been externalized from the uterus into a warm saline bath following preparation of the mother by mid-spinal transection. Analysis was restricted to focal events involving synchronous forelimb or hindlimb activity. Filmed records were examined frame-by-frame to quantify the timing of individual stroke cycles of limb movements. The degree of coordination was assessed by comparing the duration and phase of each stroke cycle by limbs within the same girdle (shoulder or pelvic). A peak in the phase values near 0.5, and complete absence of values at 0 and 1.0, indicated that limb movements in the pelvic girdle were performed in alternation. The timing of these strokes was comparable to that exhibited during swimming by postnatal rats (Bekoff & Trainer, 1979). Alternation was also evident to a reduced degree in forelimb-forelimb strokes, providing a clear demonstration of interlimb coordination as early as one day before birth. It is important to recognize that these findings, like those reported by Provine, are predicated upon a measurement of motor patterning with reference to an implicitly random process (phase values distributed uniformly between 0 and 1.0).

Although Bekoff and Lau (1980) confirmed that some of the motor activity of fetuses exhibits coordination, they concurred with earlier observers that "the vast majority of movement observed was of the type described ... as 'random' and lacking coordination." Randomness is a recurrent theme in qualitative descriptions of fetal behavior (Angulo y Gonzalez, 1932; Windle, 1944; Narayanan et al., 1971; Hamburger, 1973), yet the issue of randomness has rarely been subjected to empirical scrutiny. In our own program of research on the behavioral biology of the rat fetus, we have sought to make concepts of behavioral randomness explicit and operational (Metz, 1974). Stochastic models have been extensively employed to characterize emergent behavioral organization and to probe the age-dependent and environmental influences that contribute to the prenatal development of behavior (Smotherman & Robinson, 1986a; Robinson & Smotherman, 1987).

In this research, pregnant rats are prepared with a reversible spinal anesthetic and placed in a temperature-regulated bath containing a physiological saline solution. Individual fetuses are then directly observed through the transparent uterine wall or after delivery into the bath with or without intact embryonic membranes. Care is always taken to maintain placental attachment to the uterus and undisturbed umbilical blood circulation. These procedures provide healthy fetuses as subjects for behavioral observation for one hour or more (Smotherman et al., 1986), although typical observation sessions last 30 min or less. Fetuses observed under these conditions exhibit a diverse repertoire of motor behavior that expands from the onset of motility (about day 16 of gestation) through term (day 21.5; Smotherman & Robinson, 1986a). The fact that these measures of fetal behavior are not artifacts of the conditions of observation has been confirmed by endoscopic visualization of fetuses in vivo (Smotherman & Robinson, 1986b). Using these observational procedures, we have found that some of the spontaneous movements of rat fetuses can indeed be characterized as random. However, within a few days of the onset of motility, fetal behavior begins to exhibit nonrandom organization in temporal pattern and spatial form.

FIRST ORDER MODEL OF MOVEMENT SYNCHRONY

Many fetal investigators have noted that fetuses occasionally move several parts of the body at the same moment, a performance that seems to deny randomness and imply coordination. Simultaneous events may occur by coincidence, however. A null hypothesis of movement synchrony therefore assumes that simultaneous motion of two or more body regions (e.g., foreleg and rearleg) results from the chance association of independent, simple movements. Calculation of an expected frequency of chance association provides an alternative to comparing the incidence of synchronous movements to a different behavioral standard (as in the study of wing-wing coordination described above). This approach has been adopted in an explicit test of a stochastic model of movement synchrony in the rat fetus (Smotherman & Robinson, 1986a).

To apply this first order model, the overall probability (P) of simple movement events (acts involving just one body region, such as head, foreleg or trunk) is calculated for each subject fetus by dividing the total number of fetal movements by the number of 1-s intervals during the observation session in which fetal activity potentially could be scored. From basic probability theory, multiplying this simple probability by itself yields the probability of two independent movements occurring during the same interval (P^2). More generally, P^i gives the probability of co-occurrence of i independent events. Thus, the sum of P^i over the number of simple categories, multiplied by the number of intervals during an observation session, generates a predicted frequency of synchronous movements.

Predictions generated by the first order model accord well with the actual occurrence of motor synchrony on days 16 and 17 of gestation (Figure 1). Subsequent to day 17, however, synchronous movements become more abundant than can be accounted for by chance association. Just prior to parturition (day 21), comparison with model predictions

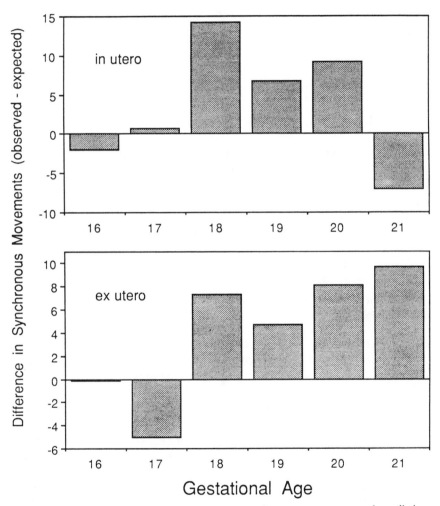

Figure 1. Discrepancy between frequencies of synchronous movement and predictions generated by the first order model of synchrony. Data are plotted as a function of gestational age for each of two micro-environments of observation (in utero and ex utero).

reveals that synchronous movements are in fact less common than should occur by random association when fetuses remain within the uterus during observation. However, when fetuses are delivered from the uterus into a warm saline bath prior to observation, taking care to preserve the integrity of umbilical blood circulation, no such reduction in synchronous movement on day 21 is apparent. We have interpreted this effect as evidence of the behavioral effects of physical restraint imposed by diminished free space within the uterus near term. The clear implication of these results is that the behavior of the rat fetus exhibits subtle organization that emerges over the last four days of gestation and exhibits sensitivity to changes that occur within the intrauterine environment (Smotherman & Robinson, 1988).

SECOND ORDER MODEL OF MOVEMENT SYNCHRONY

The first order model is sufficient to explain the simultaneous movement of several body regions from the onset of fetal motility (day 16) through day 17 of gestation. The relative abundance of synchronous movements on and after day 18, however, must be addressed by a more detailed model. A second order model has been developed to determine whether some aspects of the synchronous behavior of fetal rats after day 17 continues to be shaped by random processes (Robinson & Smotherman, 1987). Unlike the first order model, which generates the predicted total frequency of synchronous movement from the observed total frequency of fetal movement, the second order model is not dependent upon the rate of fetal activity. Instead, it focuses on the eight most common categories of synchronous movement and predicts the frequency of each category from (a) the total frequency of all synchronous movements and (b) the probability of occurrence of each category of simple movement. The second order model thus generates predictions about how behavior will be distributed among specific categories of synchronous movement. Predictions involve calculation of the probability (P_i) that a given synchronous movement includes motion of body region i. For example, the synchronous movement event foreleg-rearleg-head includes movements in three distinct body regions. P_i and its complement (which indicates the probability that a given movement does not comprise body region i) are calculated for each body region. From these probabilities, the likelihood of a movement involving regions i and j, but no other (P_{ij}), is computed as the product of P_i, P_j, and the complements of the probabilities of all other regions.

The second order model is broadly predictive of the occurrence of the focal categories of fetal movement over days 17−21 of gestation. (Because synchronous movements are almost nonexistent on day 16, the model is inapplicable at this age.) However, several categories of synchronous movement occur more frequently than can be accounted for by a simple random process (Figure 2). Noteworthy among these are the movement combinations: foreleg-rearleg, foreleg-head, and head-mouth. Other categories, such as head-rearleg, occur less often than chance association would predict. These particular linkages are intriguing because they constitute components of action patterns that assume importance during the early postnatal period. Interlimb synchrony (foreleg-rearleg) is, of course, fundamental to the development of quadrupedal locomotion, including crawling and walking. But another pattern of locomotion—punting—predominates during the first few days of postnatal life when altricial offspring are unable to support their body weight (Altman & Sudarshan, 1975).

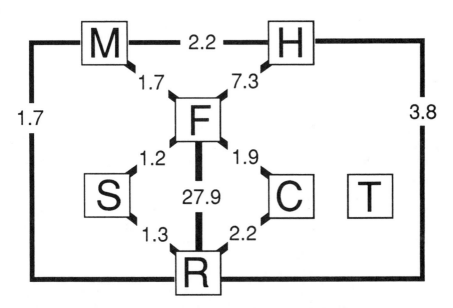

Figure 2. Diagram depicting linkage relationships between pairs of body regions on day 21 of gestation, with fetuses observed *ex utero*: M (mouth), H (head), F (foreleg), S (dorsal trunk stretch), C (ventral or lateral trunk curl), T (thoracic twitch), R (rearleg). Each line connects two regions that moved synchronously with a mean frequency exceeding 1.0 movements per 10 min. Numbers superimposed on lines show actual mean frequencies of synchronous occurrence.

Punting involves spreading the rearlegs, supporting the anterior half of the body with the head, and sweeping one foreleg laterally. The result of these coordinated movements is to pivot the pup around an anchor point provided by the rearlegs. With punting alone, neonatal rat pups are able to orient and move toward preferred objects (such as the nipple) and to maintain their position in a huddle with littermates within the nest (Alberts & Cramer, 1988). Yet if any of the three principal elements of punting were to drop out of the pattern (anchoring by the rearlegs, support by the head, propulsion by a foreleg), the whole pattern would lose its locomotor effect.

Interestingly, within 24 hours after birth, movements involving all three components (the triplet foreleg-rearleg-head) occur more often than any other category of synchronous movement. This triplet is even more in evidence if pups are mechanically supported to reduce postural, gravitational and substrate constraints on movement. The most parsimonious explanation for the postnatal appearance of this pattern is the establishment of a linkage relationship between the doublets foreleg-rearleg and foreleg-head, which predominate fetal activity late in gestation. Punting thus appears to be one example of a postnatal pattern of behavior that emerges from a hierarchy of linkage relationships established in utero.

ASYNCHRONOUS TEMPORAL PATTERNING

Synchrony is but one aspect of the temporal organization of behavior. Postnatal behavior characteristically entails fluctuations in levels of activity on multiple time scales. One aspect of temporal patterning is cyclic activity, which can be manifest on the level of circadian rhythms (see Reppert & Weaver, this volume) or cycles of much shorter periods (see Robertson, this volume). Goal-directed behavior typically exhibits non-cyclic temporal patterning as well. Events occur in bouts and higher level clusters of bouts. The existence of bouts is often invoked as a subjective appraisal from observation, but is subject to definition by more rigorous quantitative analysis. Chief among these is analysis of the length of time intervals between successive behavioral events.

If the occurrence of a particular event is independent of the time of occurrence of events that preceded it, then the cumulative distribution of inter-event interval lengths will be described by a log survivor (negative exponential) function (Fagen & Young, 1978). When such a distribution is plotted on a semilogarithmic graph, with the ordinate displaying the log of the number of intervals of length greater than t, the data fall along a straight line (Figure 3). Behavioral data that are well described by a

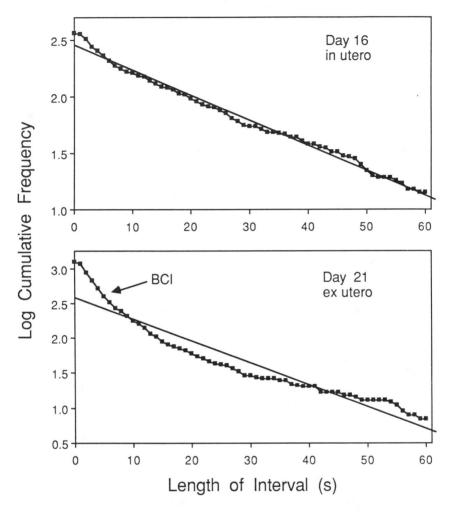

Figure 3. Representative log survivor curves of intervals between successive fetal movements on days 16 (in utero) and 21 (ex utero). Points are superimposed on the best-fitting negative exponential function as determined by a recursive algorithm. The objectively determined bout criterion interval is indicated on the graph for day 21 fetuses.

log survivor function can be considered as point events with a constant probability of occurrence in a given time interval.

We have employed log survivor analysis of interval length to determine whether asynchronous temporal patterning is evident in the activity of rat fetuses (Smotherman & Robinson, 1986a). In general, fetuses on day 16 of gestation exhibit movements that are temporally independent of one another. At later ages, short inter-event intervals (0–5 s) become more common than can be explained by random production of movements in time. Deviation from the log survivor model is most pronounced on day 21, when the number of short intervals exceeds predictions by more than 150%.

The existence of bout structure in the behavior of fetuses on days 17–21 has been confirmed through the use of an objective method for identifying a bout criterion interval. Successive events separated by an interval less than the bout criterion are defined as belonging to the same bout. The bout criterion is often determined subjectively by estimating the point on the log survivor curve where the slope changes most abruptly (Fagen & Young, 1978). But the bout criterion can be determined objectively through the application of a recursive algorithm (Machlis, 1977). The algorithm consists of six steps: (a) The bout criterion interval is initially set at 0 s. (b) The cumulative distribution of all intervals exceeding the bout criterion is tabulated. (c) A best-fitting log survivor function is determined through successive approximations to a negative exponential distribution; (d) the observed distribution is statistically compared to the exponential distribution with a nonparametric goodness-of-fit test. (e) If the null hypothesis cannot be rejected, then the procedure ends and the current bout criterion interval is adopted. (f) If the observed distribution is found to significantly differ from the theoretical distribution, then the bout criterion is incremented by one and steps (b) through (f) repeated.

Machlis (1977) developed this procedure for the temporal analysis of bout structure in the pecking behavior of chicks. She found not only that pecks tend to occur within objective bouts, but that bouts occur in higher units of clustering, which she termed superbouts. Other investigators have found that, in different applications, an objective bout criterion is problematic to determine (Slater & Lester, 1982). These facts argue that the procedure is robust in identifying bouts when bout structure exists and breaks down when the temporal organization of behavior is not well described by the concept of events clustering in bouts. When this procedure is applied to the activity of rat fetuses, an objective bout criterion is not apparent on day 16, but can be determined within the narrow range of 2–5 s in all comparisons conducted between days 17 and 21 of gestation. Although the deviation from a random temporal distribution is more pronounced later in gestation (especially on day 21), the bout criterion interval remains consistently less than 6 s. This finding may be interpreted as particularly strong evidence that fetal activity is randomly distributed on day 16 but exhibits an increasing tendency to cluster in bouts on day 17 and thereafter.

SEQUENTIAL BEHAVIORAL STRUCTURE

Postnatal behavior, and goal-directed behavior in particular, is often organized in functional sequences. Much can be inferred of underlying mechanisms controlling behavior from sequential analysis (Hailman & Sustare, 1973; Fentress & McLeod, 1986). Most analyses have assumed a Markov model in dealing with sequential relationships (Fagen & Young, 1978; Bakeman & Gottman, 1987). A Markov process exists when a system can express any of a finite number of discrete states, but knowledge of the immediately preceding state completely determines the next state to occur. More useful for biologists, a Markov chain broadens the concept of Markov process to allow for a stochastic, rather than deterministic, relationship between successive states.

To apply a Markov sequential model to behavior, the frequency of all possible ordered pairs of behavioral events is tallied in a transition matrix. Obviously, the size of this table increases as the square of the number of behavioral categories, so careful thought should be devoted to the manner in which the stream of behavior is parsed into discrete, operationally defined categories (see Fentress & McLeod, this volume). The pattern of transitions between categories can be expressed as joint probabilities (i.e., the probability of the sequence of event i followed by event j) or, which is often more informative, as contingent probabilities (the probability, given the immediate occurrence of event i, that event j will occur next).

Several methods are available for interpreting the information in a transition matrix (Bakeman & Gottman, 1987). It is possible to determine the statistical significance of individual transitions between focal categories of behavior or to test whether the distribution of transitions in the entire table deviates from a stochastic model of independence. The most common model for generating expected frequencies of transition is that used in the familiar Chi-square test: row and column totals are used to calculate the expected frequency in each cell of the matrix. When applied to a matrix of two-event transitions for rat fetuses, the observed sequential pattern is nearly exactly described by a stochastic model on day 16 of gestation. On days 17 through 21, however, observed patterns of sequential transition differ greatly from the random model.

The developmental change in sequential structure implied by this analysis can be more precisely described through the mathematics of formal information theory (Shannon & Weaver, 1949). The logic of using information measures to interpret sequential data is well discussed by Hailman (1977). Briefly, information theory provides a quantitative means for expressing the total amount of uncertainty or entropy in a closed system. H_0, the maximum entropy of a system, is defined solely in terms of the number of states a system can occupy; in behavioral analysis $H_0 = \log_2 N$, where N is the number of discrete behavioral categories. Entropy is expressed in bits per event, representing the number of dichotomous guesses required on average to specify an event or sequence of events. The entropy of a real system will equal H_0 when all categories of behavior exhibit the same probability of occurrence. If simple event probabilities (P_i) are not equal, then the overall entropy of the system will be described by the more general expression:

$$H_1 = \sum_{i=1}^{N} P_i(-\log_2 P_i)$$

Similarly, the entropy of the system described at the level of transitions between pairs of events (H_2) is calculated as the weighted average of the entropies for each row of the matrix. When the observed frequencies in a transition matrix are completely described by row and column totals (meaning that all events are sequentially independent), $H_1 = H_2$.

With the tools of information theory, it is possible to describe changes in the overall sequential organization of fetal behavior (Figure 4). The difference in entropy (H_0 through H_2) represents the amount of information

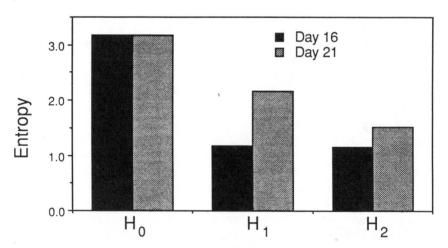

Figure 4. Information gain (bits/event) between progressively more complicated stochastic models of sequential patterning of fetal behavior. Data are presented for fetuses on gestational days 16 (*in utero*) and 21 (*ex utero*).

gained by progressing to successively more complicated levels of description. On day 16 of gestation, the greatest amount of information is gained between H_0 and H_1; at this age fetal behavior exhibits low diversity, with a few categories of movement occurring much more frequently than all others, and with almost no sequential structure. Between days 17 and 19, some information is gained between H_1 and H_2, indicating that sequential organization is beginning to emerge. Closer inspection of patterns of transition suggests that much of this structure is due to self-recursion. In other words, each category of behavior tends to follow itself in a sequence. Another important pattern that occurs at these ages is shared component transition: categories consisting of simple movement events (e.g. foreleg) tend to occur just before or after categories of synchronous movement that comprise the same kind of simple movement (e.g. foreleg and rearleg). This is perhaps not surprising, as the results of the analysis of synchronous movement indicate that specific linkages between simple movements are in the process of crystallizing as discrete categories during this time.

On gestational days 20 and 21, however, much less of the overall sequential structure can be accounted for by shared component transitions. The information gain between H_1 and H_2 is large relative to the information between H_0 and H_1. This relationship is the defining feature of a semi-Markov process (Hailman, 1977) and is characteristic of most postnatal behavior that has been described by sequential analysis. These findings clearly indicate that by late in gestation fetal behavior exhibits sequential organization. This serial patterning occurs at the same time that discrete categories of synchronous movement can be discerned (Robinson & Smotherman, 1987), bout structure becomes more pronounced, and the behavioral repertoire of the fetus expands in overall diversity (Smotherman & Robinson, 1986a). Extension of this method of sequential analysis to include pairs of events separated by intervening events (lag analysis; Bakeman & Gottman, 1987) and grouping movements into operationally delimited contiguous sets are providing additional evidence that the behavior of fetal rats becomes more contingent upon immediately preceding behavior and begins to exhibit state-like organization prior to birth (Smotherman & Robinson, 1987a).

CHANCE IN PRENATAL BEHAVIORAL DEVELOPMENT

As these analyses of movement synchrony, asynchronous temporal patterning and sequential structure suggest, random processes are likely to be fundamentally important in the early ontogeny of behavior. Before complex behavioral patterns can be expressed, the immature organism must establish physical and neural connections between the effectors involved in the action. It is possible that the physical wiring of this connectivity may be accomplished passively with respect to behavior. That is, as efferent and afferent neural fibers grow out from the CNS to establish connections with their targets a control network is established. But it is now apparent that there is a considerable overproduction of these fibers and synapses and that much of subsequent neural development consists of the selective attrition of redundant and superfluous connections through neuronal cell death. This sculpting process of neural development is promoted by function of the end organs—muscles and sense organs—and can be suspended if function is interrupted (Oppenheim, 1981; Hofer, this volume).

If behavior participates in shaping the formation of the nervous system that controls it, what is responsible for imposing pattern on behavior before the nervous system is completely formed? This question distorts the reality of embryological development somewhat, because the nervous system is certainly functional at the time of the earliest fetal movements (Hamburger, 1973; Bekoff, 1981) and there is no evidence, in mammals at least, for a preneurogenic period of motility. But it is a question that should be addressed nonetheless, as it relates directly to the problem of self-organization. The informational diversity of patterned behavior, which is now known to exist prenatally (Smotherman & Robinson, 1987b), is not present in the nervous system at the onset of fetal motility. Therefore, behavioral patterning is an emergent phenomenon whose explanation must be sought in the dynamics of a developing system and not as a passive product of anatomical maturation (Oyama, 1985).

A full answer to this question is not available, but it seems necessary that random processes are an important aspect of the self-organization of prenatal behavioral development. Just as there is an overproduction of neurons and synapses during early neural outgrowth, there appears to be an overproduction of certain aspects of behavior during the prenatal and early postnatal period (Marler & Peters, 1982). The initial randomness in movement synchrony, temporal organization and sequential structure that is evident during the first few days of fetal movement (e.g., days 16–17) give way to behavioral organization as successive levels of pattern emerge. It is reasonable to expect that selective attrition of neural structures higher in the hierarchy of control are at the root of this emergent pattern. But without production there would be nothing to select. Random production of seemingly organized activity, such as the chance synchrony of simple movements and random transition between behavioral categories, provides the stuff from which the patterning that is so evident in species-typical action patterns and goal-directed behavior in general is sculpted.

THE CHUNK MODEL OF EARLY BEHAVIORAL DEVELOPMENT

The following verbal model is offered as a working hypothesis of the rules governing the earliest phases of behavioral development. The first movements of the fetus consist of simple elements, comprising one or more motor units acting to produce motion in a single vector. When new elements appear during development their occurrence is spontaneous and random with respect to time, serial relationship and spatial patterning. The chance association of randomly generated simple movements provides afferent feedback that facilitates the selective reinforcement of linkage relationships. In effect, simple motor elements become merged as chunks. As chunks are established, spontaneity is transferred to superior levels of hierarchical control. In this way behavioral organization emerges within chunks, but motor activity continues to be governed by chance at the highest levels of chunking (the incomplete hierarchy). As the depth of linkage increases during development, spontaneity is gradually lost at inferior levels, so non-linked elements and low-level chunks eventually cease to be expressed (although they may not disappear entirely from the repertoire; see Bekoff & Kauer, 1984). In this way, novel patterns of behavior can become established in the repertoire. An example of this process may be seen in interlimb synchronization, in which the linkage of foreleg and rearleg emerges from a background of randomly associated limb movements. As a network of chunks and their constituent elements becomes established, coordinated behavior begins to assume the charac-teristics of a dynamic system. It is at this time, toward the end of the prenatal period and the beginning of postnatal life, that concepts of synergism can be usefully applied to the control and development of motor behavior (Fentress, 1984; Thelen et al., 1987).

A principal prediction from this working model is the existence of behavioral elements or chunks that exist for a period of time during the early development and later disappear from the repertoire. Such Transient Ontogenetic Behavior (TOB for short) may be viewed as a form of ontogenetic adaptation (Oppenheim 1984). The existence of TOBs is important in early behavioral development in the same way that scaffolding is important in the construction of an arch. The individual blocks of the arch cannot be set in place without supporting structures, but when the arch is complete the support system can be removed. Similarly, TOBs may develop and persist for a brief time to facilitate the elaboration of an organized behavioral network, but disappear after the network is formed. This conception of TOBs as behavioral scaffolding may apply regard-less of whether the network is preformed in the sense of a neural plan (analogous to the templates that may be involved in the ontogeny of bird song; Bottjer & Arnold, 1986) or emergent as a product of self-organization (as in the complex and organized nests that are constructed by uncoordinated activities of social insects; Wilson, 1971).

Is there currently any evidence for the existence of TOBs? Although little effort has been made to date to identify TOBs in prenatal behavioral development, it appears that one important example has been known since the early research of Preyer (1885). Fetal movements are spontaneous. Unambiguous demonstrations exist for avian embryos that such spontaneity is neurogenic and is produced by central pattern generators located within the spinal cord (Provine, 1973; Bekoff, 1981). If neural communication within the spinal cord of mammalian fetuses is interrupted by transection at the cervical or high thoracic level, spontaneous motor activity persists posterior to the site of transection (Smotherman & Robinson, unpublished data). Yet severing the spinal cord in adults produces paralysis. Because local spontaneity of motor activity is an important aspect of fetal behavior, but disappears after higher levels of neural control are established, it may be the best example of transient ontogenetic behavior.

CONCLUDING REMARKS

We hope in this essay to have persuaded the reader that there is a continuing role for the direct observation of behavior in understanding prenatal behavioral development. As Keith Nelson argued over a decade ago (1973), there is a future for the holistic study of behavior. Understanding behavioral development during the prenatal period, like the postnatal period, will continue to demand analysis at a behavioral level. Problems of pattern and process in prenatal behavior are unlikely to be solved in the short term, and may be intrinsically insoluble, if addressed solely from reductionistic perspectives. Prenatal behavior seems to exhibit characteristics of a self-organizing system. In general, this organization takes the form of a transition from randomness to increasing depth of structural relationship.

Application of quantitative concepts, especially those of stochastic models (Metz, 1974) and hierarchical organization (Fentress, 1983), look to be especially useful in revealing empirically consistent rules of prenatal behavioral development. At the least, the testing of stochastic models requires that fetal behavior be observed carefully, recorded accurately and described in quantitative terms, thus providing an objective basis for comparison and description of changes in overall behavioral organization during ontogeny. More importantly, the wider adoption of stochastic modelling techniques may generate and test hypotheses concerning underlying processes of early behavioral development. Once specific research hypotheses have been generated from observational study, they can be explicitly tested in traditional experimental situations. For example, models of movement synchrony and serial organization can lead to specific predictions about the effects of deafferentation or neural transection experiments. Similarly, the inference of behavioral states from sequential analysis of spontaneous fetal movement suggests that fetuses may respond to stimulation differently as a function of immediately preceding behavior (Smotherman & Robinson, 1987a). Quantitative observation is a research strategy that is independent from but complementary to the neuroethological approach to understanding the prenatal roots of complex behavior.

Acknowledgements

This research is supported by grant HD 16102−06 and Research Career Development Award HD 00719−01 to WPS.

References

Alberts, J. R., & Cramer, C. (1988). Ecology and experience: sources of means and meaning in developmental change. In E. M. Blass (ed.), *Handbook of behavioral neurobiology, Vol. 9, behavioral ecology and developmental psychobiology* (pp. 1−39). New York: Plenum.

Altman, J., & Sudarshan, K. (1975). Postnatal development of locomotion in the laboratory rat. *Animal Behavior, 23*, 896−920.

Angulo y Gonzalez, A. W. (1932). The prenatal development of behavior in the albino rat. *Journal of Comparative Neurology, 55*, 395−442.

Bakeman, R., & Gottman, J. M. (1987). *Observing Interaction: An Introduction to Sequential Analysis.* Cambridge: Cambridge Univ. Press.

Bekoff, A. (1981). Embryonic development of the neural circuitry underlying motor coordination. In W. M. Cowan (Ed.), *Studies in developmental neurobiology: essays in honor of Viktor Hamburger* (pp. 134−170). New York: Oxford Univ. Press.

Bekoff, A., & Kauer, J. A. (1984). Neural control of hatching: fate of the pattern generator for the leg movements of hatching in post-hatching chicks. *Journal of Neuroscience, 4*, 2659−2666.

Bekoff, A., & Lau, B. (1980). Interlimb coordination in 20−day−old rat fetuses. *Journal of Experimental Zoology, 214*, 173−175.

Bottjer, S. W., & Arnold, A. P. (1986). The ontogeny of vocal learning in songbirds. In E. M. Blass (Ed.), *Handbook of behavioral neurobiology, vol. 8, developmental psychobiology and developmental neurobiology* (pp. 129−161). New York: Plenum.

Coghill, G. E. (1929). *Anatomy and the Problem of Behavior.* Cambridge: Cambridge Univ. Press.

Colgan, P. W. (Ed.). (1978). *Quantitative Ethology.* New York: Wiley.

Dawkins, R. (1976). Hierarchical organisation: a candidate principle for ethology. In P. P. G. Bateson & R. A. Hinde (Eds.), *Growing points in ethology* (pp. 7–54). Cambridge: Cambridge Univ. Press.

Fagen, R. M., & Young, D. Y. (1978). Temporal patterns of behaviors: durations, intervals, latencies and sequences. In P. W. Colgan (Ed.), *Quantitative ethology* (pp. 79–114). New York: Wiley.

Fentress, J. C. (1983). Ethological models of hierarchy and patterning of species-specific behavior. In E. Satinoff & P. Teitelbaum (Eds.), *Handbook of behavioral neurobiology, vol. 6, motivation* (pp. 185–234). New York: Plenum.

Fentress, J. C. (1984). The development of coordination. *Journal of Motor Behavior, 16,* 99–134.

Fentress, J. C., & McLeod, P. J. (1986). Motor patterns in development. In E. M. Blass (Ed.), *Handbook of behavioral neurobiology, vol. 8, Developmental psychobiology and developmental neurobiology* (pp. 35–97). New York: Plenum.

Hailman, J. P. (1977). *Optical Signals: Animal Communication and Light.* Bloomington: Indiana University Press.

Hailman, J. P., & Sustare, B. D. (1973). What a stuffed toy tells a stuffed shirt. *Bioscience, 23,* 644–651.

Hamburger, V. (1973). Anatomical and physiological basis of embryonic motility in birds and mammals. In G. Gottlieb (Ed.), *Behavioral Embryology* (pp. 51–76). New York: Academic Press.

Kugler, P. N., Kelso, J. A. S., & Turvey, M. T. (1982). Information, coordination and control in motor skill development. In J. A. S. Kelso & J. E. Clark (Eds.), *The development of movement control and coordination* (pp. 1–78). New York: Wiley.

Machlis, L. (1977). An analysis of the temporal patterning of pecking in chicks. *Behaviour, 63,* 1–70.

Marler, P., & Peters, S. (1982). Developmental overproduction and selective attrition: new processes in the epigenesis of birdsong. *Developmental Psychobiology, 15,* 369–378.

Martin, P., & Bateson, P. (1986). *Measuring behaviour.* Cambridge: Cambridge University Press.

Metz, H. (1974). Stochastic models for the temporal fine structure of behaviour sequences. In D. J. McFarland (Ed.), *Motivational control systems analysis* (pp. 5–86). New York: Academic Press.

Narayanan, C. H., Fox, M. W., & Hamburger, V. (1971). Prenatal development of spontaneous and evoked activity in the rat. *Behaviour, 40,* 100–134.

Nelson, K. (1973). Does the holistic study of behavior have a future? In P. P. G. Bateson & P. H. Klopfer (Eds.), *Perspectives in ethology* (pp. 281–328). New York: Plenum.

Oppenheim, R. W. (1981). Neuronal cell death and some related regressive phenomena during neurogenesis: a selective historical review and progress report. In W. M. Cowan (Ed.), *Studies in developmental neurobiology: essays in honor of Viktor Hamburger* (pp. 74–133). New York: Oxford University Press.

Oppenheim R. W. (1984). Ontogenetic adaptations in neural development: toward a more 'ecological' developmental psychobiology. In H. F. R. Prechtl (Ed.), *Continuity of neural functions from prenatal to postnatal life* (pp. 16–30). Philadelphia: Lippincott.

Oyama, S. (1985). *The Ontogeny of Information: Developmental Systems and Evolution.* Cambridge: Cambridge University Press.

Preyer, W. (1885). *Specielle Physiologie des Embryo. Untersuchungen über die Lebenserscheinungen vor der Geburt.* Leipzig: Grieben.

Provine, R. R. (1973). Neurophysiological aspects of behavior development in the chick embryo. In G. Gottlieb (Ed.), *Behavioral embryology* (pp. 77–102). New York: Academic Press.

Provine, R. R. (1980). Development of between-limb movement synchronization in the chick embryo. *Developmental Psychobiology, 13*, 151–163.

Robinson, S. R., & Smotherman, W. P. (1987). Environmental determinants of behaviour in the rat fetus. II. The emergence of synchronous movement. *Animal Behaviour, 35*, 1652–1662.

Sackett, G. P. (Ed.). (1978). *Observing Behavior, vol. 2: Data Collection and Analysis Methods*. Baltimore: University Park Press.

Shannon, C. E., & Weaver, W. (1949). *The Mathematical Theory of Communication*. Urbana: University of Illinois Press.

Slater, P. J. B., & Lester, N. P. (1982). Minimising errors in splitting behaviour into bouts. *Behaviour, 79*, 153–161.

Smotherman, W. P., & Robinson, S. R. (1986a). Environmental determinants of behaviour in the rat fetus. *Animal Behaviour, 34*, 1859–1873.

Smotherman, W. P. & Robinson, S. R. (1986b). A method for endoscopic visualization of rat fetuses in situ. *Physiology & Behavior, 37*, 663–665.

Smotherman, W. P. & Robinson, S. R. (1987a). Psychobiology of fetal experience in the rat. In N. A. Krasnegor, E. M. Blass, M. A. Hofer & W. P. Smotherman (Eds.), *Perinatal development: a psychobiological perspective* (pp. 39–60). Orlando: Academic Press.

Smotherman, W. P., & Robinson, S. R. (1987b). Prenatal expression of species- typical action patterns in the rat fetus (*Rattus norvegicus*). *Journal of Comparative Psychology, 101*, 190–196.

Smotherman, W. P., & Robinson, S. R. (1988). The uterus as environment: the ecology of fetal behavior. In E. M. Blass (Ed.), *Handbook of behavioral neurobiology, vol. 9, developmental psychobiology and behavioral ecology* (pp. 149–196). New York: Plenum.

Smotherman, W. P., Robinson, S. R., & Miller, B. J. (1986). A reversible preparation for observing the behavior of fetal rats in utero: spinal anesthesia with lidocaine. *Physiology & Behavior, 37*, 57–60.

Thelen, E., Kelso, J. A. S., & Fogel, A. (1987). Self-organizing systems and infant motor development. *Developmental Review, 7*, 39–65.

Weiss, P. (1941). Self-differentiation of the basic patterns of coordination. *Comparative Psychology Monographs, 17*, 1–96.

Wilson, E. O. (1971). *The Insect Societies*. Cambridge: Harvard Univ. Press.

Windle, W. F. (1944). Genesis of somatic motor function in mammalian embryos: a synthesizing article. *Physiological Zoology, 17*, 247–261.

RESPONSE TO ENVIRONMENT

Maternal Transduction of Light-dark Information for the Fetus

Steven M. Reppert and David R. Weaver
Laboratory of Developmental Chronobiology
Children's Service
Massachusetts General Hospital
and Harvard Medical School
Boston, Massachusetts

Light has been regarded as the least likely environmental stimulus to reach the mammalian fetus (Bradley & Mistretta, 1975). However, work in this and other laboratories has shown that relevant aspects of the environmental light-dark cycle are perceived by the fetus. Interestingly, these forms of perception do not require light actually reaching the fetus; instead, they are indirect, mediated by the mother. During gestation, the mother transduces two aspects of the prenatal light-dark cycle into specific signals that are then communicated to the fetus; these two aspects of lighting are the phase (timing) of the light-dark cycle and daylength (the length of the light portion of the daily light-dark cycle). We refer to these two different forms of prenatal communication as (a) maternal-fetal communication of circadian phase and (b) maternal-fetal communication of daylength, respectively. In this chapter, we discuss the studies elucidating these two forms of maternal-fetal communication and highlight several experimental issues yet to be resolved.

INFLUENCE OF LIGHT ON THE CIRCADIAN TIMING SYSTEM

In adults, physiological effects of the phase and daylength aspects of the light-dark cycle are mediated by the "circadian timing system." This system is necessary for the generation, regulation and expression of circadian rhythms and is composed of a circadian pacemaker or biological clock and its input and output pathways (Fig. 1). The phase of the light-dark cycle synchronizes (entrains) the circadian pacemaker to the 24-hr period. This allows for the expression of circadian rhythms in the proper

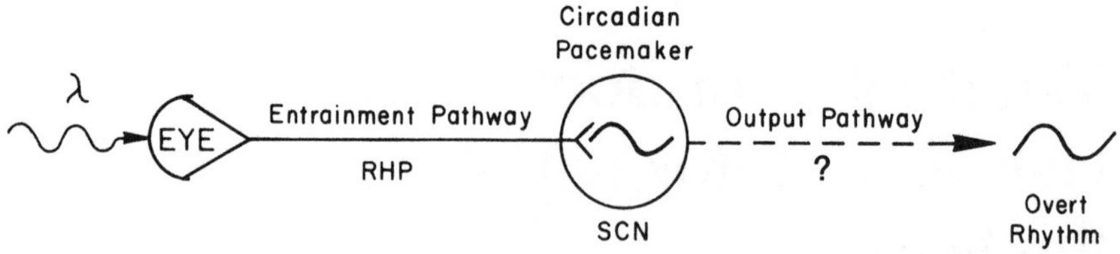

Figure 1. Major components of the mammalian circadian timing system. RHT, retinohypo-thalamic pathway; SCN, suprachiasmatic nuclei.

temporal relationship to each other and to the 24-hr day. Daylength acts through the circadian timing system to provide seasonally breeding species with information about the time of year. This seasonal information enables them to anticipate seasonal changes in the environment and to vary aspects of their physiology, such as reproduction and body weight, appropriately.

The vast majority of evidence suggests that the suprachiasmatic nuclei (SCN) of the anterior hypothalamus function as a circadian pacemaker for the circadian timing system of mammals (Moore, 1983). A direct retinohypothalamic tract transmits photic information for the circadian functions of light from the retina to the SCN pacemaker. It is important to note that in altricial rodents such as rats (*Rattus norvegicus*) the offspring are born at an immature stage of development and the retino-hypothalamic pathway does not innervate the developing SCN until the postnatal period (Stanfield & Cowan, 1976). Thus, no retina-mediated effects of light on the developing circadian timing system are possible in altricial species before birth.

MATERNAL-FETAL COMMUNICATION OF CIRCADIAN PHASE

A Biological Clock is Oscillating in the Fetus

In rats, circadian rhythmicity in biological variables is a postnatal event, with most behavioral and hormonal rhythms not expressed until the second or third weeks of life (for review see Reppert, 1987). Deguchi (1975) was the first to suggest that a biological clock might be functioning prior to the time that circadian rhythms are overtly expressed. To demonstrate influences on the developing biological clock that occur before the overt expression of rhythmicity, he determined the phase of a rhythm monitored under constant conditions during the postnatal period to infer the phase of the biological clock at earlier developmental stages. His findings suggested that a circadian clock is oscillating at or before birth and that its phase is coordinated with the dam. Since Deguchi's report, several investigators (Davis & Gorski, 1986; Fuchs & Moore, 1980; Hiroshige, Honma, & Watanabe, 1982; Pratt & Goldman, 1986; Reppert, Coleman, Heath, & Swedlow, 1984; Reppert & Schwartz, 1983; Reppert & Schwartz, 1984b; Takahashi & Deguchi, 1983; Viswanathan & Chandrashekaran, 1984; Weaver & Reppert, 1987) have used a variety of pre- and postnatal rhythms to confirm the perinatal coordination of maternal and pup rhythms in several species (Table 1).

TABLE 1

Perinatal communication of circadian phase in mammals

Species	Rhythm examined
Rat	Pup NAT activity
(*Rattus norvegicus*)	Pup drinking behavior
	Pup locomotor activity
	Pup serum corticosterone
	Pup SCN metabolic activity
	Fetal SCN metabolic activity
	Fetal SCN vasopressin mRNA
Syrian hamster	Pup locomotor activity
(*Mesocricetus auratus*)	
Djungarian hamster	Pup locomotor activity
(*Phodopus sungorus*)	
Spiny mouse	Pup locomotor activity
(*Acomys cahirinus*)	Fetal SCN metabolic activity
Field mouse	Pup locomotor activity
(*Mus booduga*)	
Squirrel monkey	Fetal SCN metabolic activity
(*Saimiri sciureus*)	

NAT; pineal N-acetyltransferase   SCN; suprachiasmatic nuclei

Because of the possibility that some rhythmic aspect of the birth process itself could start or set the timing of the developing clock, postnatal paradigms cannot conclusively show that a circadian clock actually functions in utero. Demonstrating prenatal function of the circadian clock requires a method than can measure an intrinsic, functionally relevant property of the clock itself. A method proven useful for monitoring the oscillatory activity of the SCN in adult rats is 2-deoxyglucose (2–DG) autoradiography (Schwartz, Davidson, & Smith, 1980; Schwartz & Gainer, 1977), which is used to determine the rates of glucose utilization (metabolic activity) of individual brain structures in vivo (Sokoloff et al., 1977).

Reppert and Schwartz (1983) successfully demonstrated a circadian rhythm of metabolic activity in the fetal rat SCN with the 2–DG technique. This study indicated that the fetal SCN show circadian variation in metabolic activity that is "in time" (coordinated) with the rhythm in the dam and with the external lighting cycle (Fig. 2). Remarkably, this fetal rhythm can be detected 2 to 3 days before birth (as early as day 19 of gestation; Reppert & Schwartz, 1984a). It is interesting to note that neurogenesis of the rat SCN occurs between days 13 and 16 of gestation (Altman & Bayer, 1978; Ifft, 1972). Immature synapses first appear in the SCN on gestational day 18 (Koritsanszky, 1981), and the vast majority of synapses appear postnatally (Lenn, Beebe, & Moore, 1977). In addition, a rhythm in SCN action potentials cannot be detected in hypothalamic slices until the end of the second postnatal week (Shibata, Liou, & Ueki, 1983). Thus, the day-night variation in SCN metabolic activity during fetal life is not dependent on a rich array of synaptic interactions or the rhythm in SCN electrical activity.

This early circadian function and its independence from synaptic activity raises several interesting questions yet to be resolved. For example, what is the nature of the cellular events underlying this early spontaneous oscillation of metabolic activity? How do neurons in the fetal SCN communicated with each other (that is, oscillate as a unit) in the absence of neural connections? Answers to these questions may provide important insights into the mechanisms underlying circadian oscillations in mammals.

Maternal Communication of Circadian Phase to the Fetal Biological Clock

The 2–DG method also has been used to show that maternal-fetal communication of circadian phase actually occurs *in utero* (Reppert & Schwartz, 1983). Blind dams were used to show that environmental lighting acts through the maternal circadian system to entrain the rhythm of fetal SCN metabolic activity; the fetal rhythm was synchronous with the circadian time of the blind mothers and not affected directly by ambient lighting.

Maternal-fetal communication of circadian phase appears to be the result of communication of some signal from dam to fetuses that results in

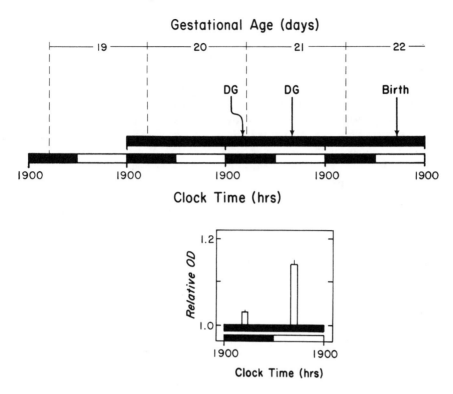

Figure 2. Deoxyglucose experiment showing that the fetal SCN manifest a day-night rhythm in metabolic activity. Four pregnant Sprague-Dawley rats were housed with lights on from 0700 to 1900h until gestational day 19, when the animals were placed in constant darkness in preparation for the deoxyglucose injection (experimental paradigm depicted in upper panel). Two animals were injected i.v. with 2−deoxy[^{14}C]glucose during the period when the lights would have normally been off (subjective night) on gestational day 20, and the other two were injected during the period when the lights would have normally been on (subjective day) on gestational day 21. At 45 min after injection, the animals were killed and four fetal brains from each pregnant animal were randomly chosen, sectioned and processed for autoradiography. The optical density (OD) of each fetal suprachiasmatic nucleus was measured and the OD of adjacent hypothalamus was used as an internal reference standard for each fetal brain. The data are thus expressed as relative OD (OD of SCN/OD of adjacent hypothalamus). Each vertical bar in the lower panel gives mean relative OD (+SEM) for the SCN of eight fetal brains. The fetal SCN exhibit a clear day-night rhythm of metabolic activity ($p<0.01$); the nuclei are metabolically active during the mother's subjective day and inactive during mother's subjective night. From Reppert, Duncan, & Goldman, 1985.

entrainment of the fetuses. The involvement of maternal circadian rhythmicity in the generation of the entraining signal(s) has been demonstrated in rats (Reppert & Schwartz, 1986a) and Syrian hamsters (*Mesocricetus auratus*; Davis & Gorski, 1983) by destroying the maternal SCN early in gestation. The fetal SCN appear to develop normally and even begin to oscillate after maternal SCN lesions, but they are no longer coordinated to the lighting conditions in the outside world or to their litter mates. These experiments indicate that the entraining signal depends on the integrity of the maternal SCN (Fig. 3a). We have recently shown that during the postnatal period, pups of SCN lesioned dams respond appropriately (entrain) to light-dark cycles despite the absence of prenatal maternal entrainment (unpublished data). Furthermore, pups from sham-operated and SCN-lesioned dams express free running rhythms with similar cycle lengths (Reppert & Schwartz, 1986a). Thus, normal circadian rhythmicity (e.g., light-dark entrainment and free running cycle length) in adulthood does not appear to require prenatal maternal entrainment.

Studies have been conducted in an attempt to identify the maternal signal(s) that communicates circadian phase to rat fetuses. Since the in utero environment provides a rich source of rhythmic hormones from the mother (e.g, prolactin, corticosterone and melatonin), studies in rats have focused on the possibility that the maternal entraining signal is a hormone. Melatonin, the principal hormone of the pineal gland, was a prime candidate for the maternal signal communicating phase information to the fetus (Reppert, 1982). There is a robust rhythm of melatonin in the maternal circulation, and because melatonin can cross the placenta (Klein, 1972; Reppert, Chez, Anderson, & Klein, 1979), a melatonin rhythm in the dam is reflected in the fetal circulation (Reppert et al., 1979; Yellon & Longo, 1987).

However, maternal pinealectomy, which eliminates measurable levels of melatonin (Lewy et al., 1980), does not abolish maternal coordination of fetal circadian phase (Reppert & Schwartz, 1986b). Furthermore, removal of the maternal adrenals, thyroid-parathyroids, pituitary, or ovaries (in separate experiments) does not abolish the clear day-night rhythm of metabolic activity in the fetal SCN when performed on or before day 7 of gestation (the time when maternal SCN lesions are disruptive). The maternal eyes, a potential source of both neural and endocrine signals, are also not necessary for the communication, since dams enucleated on day 2 of gestation synchronize the circadian clocks of their fetuses (Reppert & Schwartz, 1983).

Following maternal SCN lesions on day 7 of gestation, disruption of maternal circadian rhythms and disruption of maternal-fetal communication of circadian phase occur together. One approach to determine which

A.

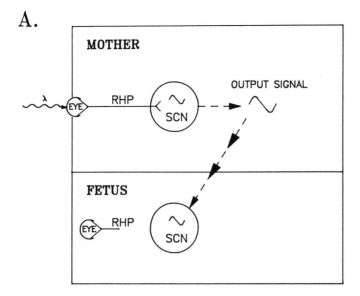

B.

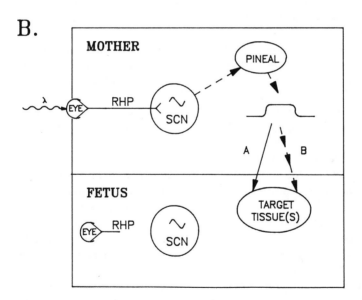

Figure 3. Conceptual models of maternal-fetal communication of circadian phase (A.) and daylength (B.). A. Light-induced neural signals are conveyed to the dam's SCN by her retinohypothalamic pathway (RHP), entraining her circadian rhythms. A maternal output signal then entrains the fetal clock at a time when the innervation of the fetal SCN by the RHP is incomplete. B. Daylength information is processed by the maternal circadian system leading to a nightly melatonin signal from the pineal gland. The melatonin signal communicates daylength to the fetus by either (a) directly acting on fetal receptive tissues or (b) initiating a cascade of hormonal events in the dam that results in some other signal reaching the fetus.

aspect of maternal rhythmicity is involved in maternal-fetal coordination is to artificially restore rhythmicity in a dam which has no endogenous rhythmicity. Normally, there is a circadian rhythm in food consumption; this rhythm is disrupted by SCN lesions (Nagai et al., 1978). Restricted access to food in SCN-lesioned rats artificially produces a rhythm in food consumption and can also induce rhythms in locomotor activity and temperature (Kreiger, Hause, & Krey, 1977; Stephan, 1981).

Using a food access restriction paradigm (food cue) in SCN-lesioned dams, our data suggest that the rhythmic ingestion of food can entrain fetuses of SCN-lesioned dams (unpublished data). Rhythmic food ingestion clearly would cause rhythmic fluctuations in nutrient levels in the blood, and this could in turn induce physiological responses to the presence of nutrients. In SCN-lesioned dams, food restriction may cause generation of a nutrient-related signal which entrains the fetuses in a manner parallel to that which occurs in intact dams. Alternatively, restricted feeding of SCN-lesioned dams leads to the generation of other rhythms (e.g., in temperature and activity) that may be involved in setting the phase of the fetuses.

Because the fetus is exposed to a multitude of maternal rhythms (behavioral rhythms, as well as hormonal), another possibility to consider is that multiple maternal rhythms act in concert to entrain the fetal biological clock. Thus, the elimination of any one of these rhythms would not be sufficient to disrupt maternal entrainment. This redundancy may explain some recent, seemingly conflicting data. As mentioned above, maternal pinealectomy does not disrupt maternal-fetal communication of circadian phase, indicating that the maternal pineal gland is not necessary for maternal entrainment. However, Davis & Mannion (1986) have presented preliminary data showing that timed injections of pharmacologic doses of melatonin into SCN-lesioned Syrian hamsters restore fetal synchrony. If this restoration of synchrony also occurs at physiologic concentrations of melatonin, it would support the redundancy hypothesis; that is, while melatonin is not necessary for synchronization, it is capable of synchronizing the fetal biological clock.

During the postnatal period, the maternal circadian system of altricial rodents continues to coordinate the timing of the developing circadian system. It appears that maternal influences during the postnatal period serve to maintain or reinforce the coordination of phase that has been established during the prenatal period. In rats, the postnatal maternal influence persists until the pup develops the potential for direct light-dark entrainment through its own eyes, at the end of the first week of life (Duncan, Banister, & Reppert, 1986).

The nature of the output signal from the maternal SCN that influences the timing of the developing circadian system during the postnatal period is also not known. It is quite possible that different output signals are used during the pre- and postnatal periods. For example, prenatal entrainment may involve rhythmic aspect of maternal physiology, such as rhythms in nutrient availability or temperature, while the postnatal effect might involve rhythmic aspects of maternal behavior, such as nursing (Hiroshige et al., 1982; Levin & Stern, 1975; Viswanathan & Chandrashekaran, 1985).

Maternal-Fetal Communication of Circadian Phase in Precocious Species

Maternal transduction appears to be the only mechanism for fetal perception of the prenatal light-dark cycle in altricial species (e.g., rats and hamsters) because the neural mechanisms for direct responsiveness to environmental lighting develop postnatally. In more precocious species, offspring are born at an advanced stage of maturation, and thus it seems likely that neural connections relaying light to the circadian timing system may be developed before birth. For example, using horseradish peroxidase histochemistry, we have demonstrated that the retinohypothalamic pathway reaches the SCN on the day of birth in spiny mice (*Acomys cahirinus*; Jacques, Weaver, & Reppert, 1987b) and guinea pigs (*Cavia porcellus*; unpublished data).

In addition to the developmental status of the fetal nervous system, the qualitative and quantitative aspects of light must be considered in determining whether light can be detected by the fetus. We have shown that a fraction of incident light is transmitted into the uterus of pregnant rats and guinea pigs (Jacques, Weaver & Reppert, 1987a). Around 500 nm, the wavelength for maximal sensitivity to the entraining influence of light (Takahashi, DeCoursey, Bauman, & Menaker, 1984), approximately 2% of incident light reaches the lumen of the uterus (Fig. 4).

We recently developed a model for examination of the potential direct photic entrainment of the fetus in precocious species using the spiny mouse. After a gestation period of 38 to 40 days, the pups are born; within hours of birth the pups are mobile, their eyes are open and auditory and olfactory senses are functional. There would appear to be little need for postnatal maternal influences on pup phase, as the pups are exposed to the environment (and presumably responsive to it) during the immediate postnatal period.

Indeed, our studies show that there is robust maternal-fetal communication of circadian phase in this precocious species, without demonstrable postnatal maternal influences on pup circadian rhythmicity (Weaver &

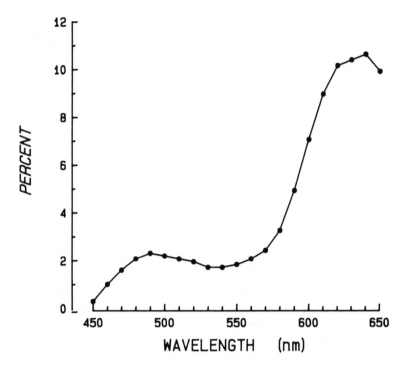

Figure 4. Transmission of light into the uterus of the guinea pig. The mean transmission level by wavelength for 6 placements (2 positions in each of 3 animals) are indicated. Modified from Jacques *et al.*, 1987.

Reppert, 1987). Furthermore, light presented at night during late fetal life is actually directly perceived by the fetus, as assessed by an increase in metabolic activity in the fetal SCN (unpublished data). Thus, it is possible that direct photic entrainment in utero augments or might even replace maternal-fetal coordination of circadian phase in precocious species. This may be particularly important in diurnal mammals, including most primate species, in which the likelihood that environmental lighting directly influences the fetus would be increased.

Potential Functions of Maternal-Fetal Communication of Circadian Phase

The presence of perinatal communication of circadian phase in several mammalian species (Table 1) suggests that this phenomenon is of adaptive value. Maternal entrainment would presumably coordinate the pups to the dam and to the environment, so that when physiological and behavioral rhythmicity later develops, the rhythms are expressed in proper relationship to one another and to the 24-h day. This allows the young animal to more easily assume its temporal niche.

If the pups were not coordinated to the environment by the mother, they might exhibit inappropriate timing of emergence from the burrow or disadvantageous behavioral patterns when they emerged (Pratt & Goldman, 1986). Furthermore, if each pup were to develop with its own rhythmicity, there would be a period of disorganization of the litter that could be detrimental to some or all members of the litter. For example, coordination of a dam's willingness to nurse and of all pups in the litter to suckle would clearly be of benefit. Circadian disorganization at the level of the individual or litter could thus threaten survival of individual pups.

Another possible function of the developing circadian clock and its entrainment during fetal life is in the initiation of parturition. This potential role of the entrained fetal SCN may be applicable to several species, because the time of day of birth is gated to the daily light-dark cycle by a circadian mechanism in a number of species (Jolly, 1972; Kaiser & Halberg, 1962; Lincoln & Porter, 1976; Rossendale & Short, 1967). If the fetuses of polytocous mammals, such as rats, are involved in the initiation of birth, then all the fetal-placental units would have to function in unison to initiate this process. Maternal entrainment of the circadian clock of each fetus may be important for providing this synchrony, and therefore may be important in the initiation of birth.

We recently examined the roles of the maternal SCN and fetal brain in the timing of birth in rats (Reppert, Henshaw, Schwartz, & Weaver 1987). First, we showed that births are more prevalent during the day, and the timing of births (relative to the time from conception) can be manipulated over a 36-h temporal "window" by altering the phase of the prenatal light-dark cycle. Next, we examined the effects of maternal SCN lesions on day 7 of gestation and found that destruction of the maternal SCN eliminated the circadian gating (i.e., preference for daytime births).

Since the fetal circadian clocks are desynchronized by maternal SCN lesions on day 7 of gestation, the fetal SCN may be a necessary component of the timing system gating parturition. Selective lesions of the SCN are very difficult if not impossible to perform in an entire litter of rat fetuses. Thus, we removed the fetal brain as a gross means of assessing the potential influence of the fetal SCN on the timing of birth. Dams of fetuses whose brains were removed on day 19 of gestation no longer exhibited a daytime preference for births; births occurred over a longer temporal window, and following a longer gestation. Importantly, the daytime preference was still present in dams with sham-operated fetuses.

These results show that the maternal SCN are necessary for the normal circadian gating of birth and are also consistent with a role for the fetal brain in this timing phenomenon. A specific role of the fetal SCN in this process still needs to be examined. Perhaps these studies should move to precocious species; the fetuses of more precocious species, such as sheep, clearly initiate the birth process (Liggins et al., 1977). Also, specific fetal output signals have been defined in sheep that are involved in parturition, as opposed to rats in which there are no such defined output signals.

MATERNAL-FETAL COMMUNICATION OF DAYLENGTH

The preceding sections have described maternal-fetal communication of circadian phase. Recent studies show that another aspect of the light-dark cycle, daylength, is also perceived by the fetus and influences development.

Photoperiodic Regulation of Reproduction

Seasonal variations in environmental conditions occur throughout temperate regions, and many animals undergo seasonal physiological changes. Daylength is the most reliable and thus most widely used indicator of season. Many species prepare for the severe climate and reduced food availability characteristic of winter by altering stores of body fat, growing a thicker and/or lighter-colored coat, and, in some species, entering hibernation or daily torpor. The most extensively studied seasonal rhythm is the annual rhythm in reproductive function; mating is generally restricted to portions of the year such that young are born in the spring and summer, when conditions are most favorable for their survival (Bronson, 1985; Karsch et al., 1984; Lincoln & Short, 1980). Many small mammals with short (< 2 months) gestation periods, including mice, voles, hamsters, rabbits, mink and ferrets, are referred to as long-day breeders, since they produce their young during favorable periods by breeding during the long days of spring and summer.

In adult long-day breeders, long daylengths stimulate or maintain reproductive function, while short photoperiods induce testicular regression in males and a cessation of estrous cyclicity in females. The influence of daylength on reproduction is blocked by pinealectomy (for reviews, see Goldman & Darrow, 1983; Karsch et al., 1984; Tamarkin, Baird, & Almeida, 1985). The involvement of melatonin as the active pineal factor mediating these effects is indicated by studies using exogenously administered melatonin (e.g., Bittman & Karsch, 1984; Goldman et al., 1982; Tamarkin, Hollister, Lefebvre, & Goldman, 1977). In several species, the duration of melatonin secretion is proportional to the length of the night, and the duration of melatonin elevation appears to be the critical parameter in mediating its effects on reproductive status (for reviews, see Goldman & Darrow, 1983; Karsch et al., 1984; Tamarkin et al., 1985).

While a great deal has been learned regarding the mechanisms for the regulation of reproduction, new concepts continue to emerge. One such concept is that an animal has a "photoperiodic history" that can strongly influence its reproductive response to photoperiod. An animal's response to a particular daylength is not absolute, but instead appears to depend in part on the preceding photoperiodic experience (Hoffmann, 1984; Rivkees, Hall, Weaver, & Reppert, 1988).

In most photoperiodic species, the timing of puberty is under photoperiodic control (Hoffman, 1978; Zucker, Johnston, & Frost, 1980). Since the developing pups respond to photoperiod prior to puberty, it is possible to use their reproductive development to study photoperiod influences early in life. In fact, it is possible to study the development of an animal's photoperiodic history by examining the rate of reproductive development in response to a test photoperiod. Studies of this type with montane voles (*Microtus montanus*; Horton, 1984) and Djungarian hamsters (*Phodopus sungorus*; Stetson, Elliott, & Goldman, 1986) have revealed an intriguing phenomenon: the developing fetus senses the daylength *in utero*, and this prenatal photoperiodic history influences the timing of puberty.

Prenatal Perception of Daylength

We have shown in our laboratory that the prenatal photoperiod influences postnatal reproductive development in Djungarian hamsters (Weaver & Reppert, 1986). This was done by exposing dams to different photoperiods during pregnancy and then rearing all the pups in the same postnatal photoperiod. Juveniles that experienced a decrease in daylength on the day of birth had significantly reduced testicular and body weights compared to those reared in the same photoperiod both pre- and postnatally (Fig. 5, upper panel). The presence of these differences between groups, which differ only in the photoperiod experienced by the dam during gestation, indicates that the prenatal photoperiod influences somatic and reproductive development.

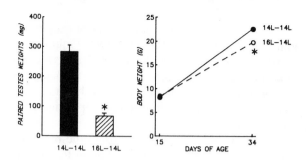

A. MALE PUPS OF INTACT DAMS

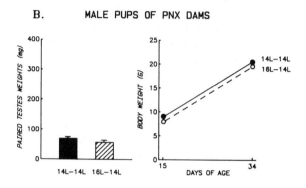

B. MALE PUPS OF PNX DAMS

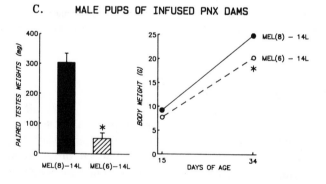

C. MALE PUPS OF INFUSED PNX DAMS

Figure 5. Mean testicular weights (left) and body weights (right) of 34-day-old Djungarian hamsters from intact dams (A)., pinealectomized dams (PNX, B.), and PNX dams receiving timed melatonin infusions during gestation (C.). Litters from dams kept in 16 h of light per day (16L) during pregnancy were shifted to 14 h of light per day (14L) on the day of birth (16L–14L group); another set of litters was kept in 14L during both the pre- and postnatal periods (14L–14L group). For the experiments of the lower panel, pinealectomized dams were infused with 50 ng of melatonin over 6-h or 8-h per night for each of a minimum of 3 nights at the end of gestation; these durations were chosen because 8-h infusions into PNX juveniles simulate 14L, while 6-h infusions simulate 16L (Carter & Goldman, 1983). In the left-hand panels, the vertical lines indicate SEMs. In the right-hand panels, SEMs are contained within the symbols for the means. Number of male pups: Intact Dam, 16L–14L, 35; Intact Dam, 14L–14L, 36; PNX Dam, 16L–14L, 17; PNX dam, 14L–14L, 17; Mel(8)–14L, 8; Mel(6)–14L, 11.* indicates P<0.01. Modified from Weaver and Reppert, 1986.

Considering the role of the pineal gland and melatonin in the photoperiodic regulation of reproduction in adult animals, we next examined the role of the maternal pineal gland in the prenatal perception of daylength. In contrast to the results from intact dams, maternal pinealectomy abolished the ability of prenatal photoperiod to alter subsequent somatic and reproductive development in the offspring (Fig. 5, middle panel). This indicates that the prenatal perception of daylength is due to reception by the fetus of a signal involving the maternal pineal gland; this phenomenon can therefore be referred to as maternal-fetal communication of daylength.

To determine whether maternal melatonin is the pineal product communicating daylength to the fetus, melatonin was infused subcutaneously into pinealectomized dams during pregnancy. Timed infusions of melatonin of various durations were delivered for the last several nights of gestation; melatonin durations (i.e., hours of infusion per night) were chosen to simulate the melatonin patterns that would be present in pineal-intact dams exposed to different photoperiods during pregnancy. Melatonin infusions were able to mimic the effects of different prenatal photoperiods on somatic and reproductive development in the offspring (Fig. 5, lower panel). There was no difference between infusions delivered during the day and at night; the important factor was infusion duration. These results show that melatonin is the pineal output communicating daylength to the fetus (Weaver & Reppert, 1986).

More recently, we have restricted the period of melatonin infusion to pinealectomized dams during gestation in order to determine when the hormone is most effective in providing the fetus with a prenatal photoperiodic history (Weaver, Keohan, & Reppert, 1987). We found that a single melatonin infusion delivered on any one night of gestation was ineffective in stimulating reproductive development of the male offspring. When two infusions were delivered on consecutive nights of gestation, however, postnatal testicular development of some litters was stimulated. The response was dependent upon the gestational age of the fetuses at the time of the infusions, with infusions delivered on any two nights between 6 and 2 nights prior to birth being most effective. The response to melatonin infusions delivered on the last two nights of gestation was dramatically smaller than the response to infusions delivered earlier, which suggests that there is a decline in the responsiveness of the fetus to melatonin. This decline may be the beginning of a period of insensitivity to melatonin that extends through the neonatal period until approximately postnatal day 15, when the pup begins to use its own melatonin pattern to measure daylength (see below).

While maternal melatonin is clearly involved in maternal-fetal communication of daylength, the mechanism by which it does so remains to be determined (Fig. 3b). Based on studies in other species, a maternal melatonin rhythm would be reflected in the fetus (Klein, 1972; Reppert et al., 1979; Yellon & Longo, 1987), and thus melatonin could act directly in the fetus to communicate daylength. Alternatively, the duration of melatonin elevation in the dam could lead to a cascade of hormonal events in the dam which results in the generation of some other signal that subsequently reaches the fetus. Our recent demonstration of putative melatonin receptors in the hypothalamus of fetal Djunganian hamsters suggests that melatonin may interact directly with the fetal brain (Weaver, Namboodiri & Reppert, 1988).

The finding that maternal melatonin communicates daylength to the fetus opens a new avenue for investigating melatonin's sites and mechanism of action. Studies of the sites and cellular mechanism by which melatonin regulates reproduction have not been successful in adult animals. Aspects of maternal-fetal communication of daylength make this an interesting system in which to address these issues. For example, the duration of melatonin treatment needed to elicit a maximal physiological response is relatively short in this system compared to adults. This developmental system provides an effective "bioassay" for characterizing various melatonin analogs. Thus, the developmental model may provide a significant tool for probing the way in which melatonin regulates reproduction and other seasonal changes.

Physiological Significance of Maternal-Fetal Communication of Daylength

Maternal-fetal communication of daylength would be of considerable value in a long-day breeder such as the Djungarian hamster. If offspring born early in the breeding season are to reproduce in the same year they are born, rapid reproductive development is necessary. Late-season offspring would be at a disadvantage, however, if they were to expend their energy rapidly reaching puberty when the end of the breeding season is approaching. Clearly, no single strategy would be appropriate for all offspring.

Daylength can be used to determine the season. Except for the solstices, any daylength occurs twice in a year, however, so the daylength at any single point in time is useless in determining the time of year. A mechanism for comparison of the daylength at two time points is needed to determine the direction of change in daylength, and to accurately determine the time of year. Maternal-fetal communication of daylength provides the fetus with one daylength measurement. Upon measuring daylength on its own during the postnatal period (beginning around postnatal day 15 (Pratt & Goldman, 1986; Tamarkin et al., 1980; Yellon, Tamarkin, & Goldman, 1985) the offspring can rapidly determine the direction of change in the daylength. In this way, maternal-fetal communication of daylength allows the pups to rapidly make the seasonally appropriate choice between preparing for the summer breeding season or preparing for winter (e.g., by altering energy metabolism and body fat stores). Interestingly, this response appears to require a "memory" of prenatal melatonin duration experienced, and a mechanism for "comparison" with melatonin durations experienced later.

Significance of Circadian Phase Communication in a Photoperiodic Species

Previous hypotheses about the possible physiological significance of maternal-fetal communication of circadian phase have centered on the value of entrainment per se in synchronizing and coordinating rhythms of the neonate with the dam (see above). Another potential value of perinatal entrainment is that it better prepares the neonate to respond to environmental cues that communicate daylength (Pratt & Goldman, 1986). For example, if pups were out of phase with the environment on first emerging from the burrow, their melatonin rhythm might be distorted for several days until it becomes fully entrained by the light-dark cycle. This distorted melatonin pattern would be inappropriate in providing daylength information. Prenatal entrainment may therefore be a physiologically important mechanism which helps photoperiodic animals accurately measure daylength immediately on emergence from the burrow, allowing rapid, appropriate determination of season.

PROSPECTUS

We have described in this chapter two novel and physiologically relevant forms of maternal-fetal communication (circadian phase and daylength). One impact of this line of investigation is that it makes us reconsider the sensory world of the fetus. The dam has typically been thought of as a protective barrier, shielding her offspring from the environment. Stimuli such as sound and light reach the fetus through maternal tissues via passive conduction. We now know that the dam tranduces sensory information for the fetus, taking a much more active role in controlling the fetus's sensory environment. Remarkably, the fetus responds to maternal signals that communicate lighting information at a time when it is incapable of directly detecting light. Maternal transduction provides the fetus with environmental information critical for normal development. This information also facilitates the transition from the uterus to life outside the womb.

Acknowledgments

Supported by March of Dimes Basic Research Grant 1−945 and Public Health Service Grant HD14427. S. M. Reppert is an Established Investigator of the American Heart Association.

References

Altman, J., & Bayer, S. A. (1978). Development of the diencephalon in the rat. I. Autoradiographic study of the time of origin and settling patterns of neurons of the hypothalamus. *Journal of Comparative Neurology, 182*, 945−972.

Bittman, E. L., & Karsch, F. J. (1984). Nightly duration of melatonin secretion determines the reproductive response to inhibitory day length in the ewe. *Biology of Reproduction, 30*, 585−593.

Bradley, R. M., & Mistretta, C. M. (1975). Fetal sensory receptors. *Physiological Reviews, 55*, 352−382.

Bronson, F. H. (1985). Mammalian reproduction: an ecological perspective. *Biology of Reproduction, 32*, 1−26.

Carter, D. S., & Goldman, B. D. (1983). Antigonadal effects of timed melatonin infusions in pinealectomized male Djungarian hamsters (*Phodopus sungorus sungorus*): Duration is the critical parameter. *Endocrinology, 113*, 1261−1267.

Davis, F. C., & Gorski, R. A. (1983). Entrainment of circadian rhythms in utero: role of the maternal suprachiasmatic nucleus. *Society for Neuroscience Abstracts, 9*, 625.

Davis, F. C., & Gorski, R. A. (1986). Development of hamster circadian rhythms II. Prenatal entrainment of the pacemaker. *Journal of Biological Rhythms, 1*, 77−85.

Davis, F. C., & Mannion, J. (1986). Melatonin during gestation affects the phase of postnatal circadian rhythms in hamsters. *Society for Neuroscience Abstracts, 12*, 212.

Deguchi, T. (1975). Ontogenesis of a biological clock for serotonin:acetyl coenzyme A N-acetyltransferase in the pineal gland of rat. *Proceedings of the National Academy of Sciences USA, 72*, 2914−2920.

Duncan, M. J., Banister, M. J., & Reppert, S. M. (1986). Developmental appearance of light-dark entrainment in the rat. *Brain Research, 369*, 326−330.

Fuchs, J. L., & Moore, R. Y. (1980). Development of circadian rhythmicity and light responsiveness in the rat suprachiasmatic nucleus. A study using 2-deoxy-$(1-^{14}C)$ glucose method. *Proceedings of the National Academy of Sciences USA, 77*, 1204−1208.

Goldman, B. D., Carter, D. S. Hall, V. D., Roychoudhury, P., & Yellon, S. M. (1982). Physiology of melatonin in three hamster species. In D. C. Klein (Ed.), *Melatonin Rhythm Generating System − Developmental Aspects* (pp. 201−231). Basel: Karger.

Goldman, B. D., & Darrow, J. M. (1983). The pineal gland and mammalian photoperiodism. *Neuroendocrinology, 73*, 386−396.

Hiroshige, T., Honma, K., & Watanabe, K. (1982). Prenatal onset and maternal modifications of the circadian rhythm of plasma corticosterone in blind infantile rats. *Journal of Physiology (Cambridge)*, *325*, 521–532.

Hoffmann, K. (1978). Effects of short photoperiod on puberty, growth and moult in the Djungarian hamster (*Phodopus sungorus*). *Journal of Reproduction and Fertility*, *54*, 29–35.

Hoffmann, K. (1984). Photoperiodic reaction in the Djungarian hamster is influenced by previous light history. *Biology of Reproduction*, *34* (Suppliment 1), 55.

Horton, T. H. (1984). Growth and reproductive development in *Microtus montanus* is affected by the prenatal photoperiod. *Biology of Reproduction*, *31*, 499–504.

Ifft, J. D. (1972). An autoradiographic study of the time of final division of neurons in rat hypothalamic nuclei. *Journal of Comparative Neurology*, *144*, 193–204.

Jacques, S. L., Weaver, D. R., & Reppert, S. M. (1987a). Penetration of light into the uterus of pregnant mammals. *Photochemistry and Photobiology*, *45*, 637–641.

Jacques, S. L., Weaver, D. R., & Reppert, S. M. (1987b). Precocious spiny mice as a model to assess the potential for retina-mediated light perception in utero. *Society for Neuroscience Abstracts 13*, 864.

Jolly, A. (1972). Hour of birth in primates and man. *Folia Primatologica*, *18*, 108–121.

Kaiser, I. H., & Halberg, F. (1962). Circadian periodic aspects of birth. *Annals of the New York Academy of Sciences*, *98*, 1056–1068.

Karsch, F. J., Bittman, E. L., Foster, D. L., Goodman, R. L., Legan, S. J., & Robinson, J. E. (1984). Neuroendocrine basis of seasonal reproduction. *Recent Progress in Hormone Research*, *40*, 185–232.

Klein, D. C. (1972). Evidence for the placental transfer of 3H-acetyl-melatonin. *Nature (New Biology)*, *237*, 117–118.

Koritsanszky, S. (1981). Fetal and early postnatal cyto- and synaptogenesis in the suprachiasmatic nucleus of the rat hypothalamus. *Acta Morphologica Academiae Scientiarum Hungaricae (Budapest)*, *29*, 227–239.

Kreiger, D. T., Hause, L., & Krey, L. C. (1977). Suprachiasmatic nuclear lesions do not abolish food-shifted circadian adrenal and temperature rhythmicity. *Science*, *197*, 398–399.

Lenn, N. J., Beebe, B., & Moore, R. Y. (1977). Postnatal development of the suprachiasmatic nucleus of the rat. *Cell and Tissue Research*, *178*, 463–475.

Levin, R. & Stern, J. M. (1975). Maternal influences on ontogeny of suckling and feeding rhythms in the rat. *Journal of Comparative and Physiological Psychology*, *89*, 711–721.

Lewy, A. J., Tetsuo, M., Markey, S. P., Goodwin, F. K., & Kopin, I. J. (1980). Pinealectomy abolishes plasma melatonin in the rat. *Journal of Clinical Endocrinology and Metabolism*, *50*, 204–207.

Liggins, G. C., Fairclough, R. J., Grieves, S. A., Forster, C. S., & Knox, B. S. (1977). Parturition in the sheep. In J. Knight & M. O'Connor, M. (Eds.), *Ciba Foundation Symposium*, *47*, 5–30.

Lincoln, D. W., & Porter, D. G. (1976). Timing of the photoperiod and the hour of birth in rats. *Nature (London)*, *260*, 780–781.

Lincoln, G. A., & Short, R. V. (1980). Seasonal breeding: nature's contraceptive. *Recent Progress in Hormone Research*, *36*, 1–43.

Moore, R. Y. (1983). Organization and function of a central nervous system circadian oscillator: the suprachiasmatic hypothalamic nucleus. *Federation Proceedings*, *42*, 2783–2789.

Nagai, K., Nishino, T., Nakagawa, H., Nakamura, S., & Fukuda, Y. (1978). Effect of bilateral lesions of the suprachiasmatic nuclei on the circadian rhythms of food intake. *Brain Research*, *142*, 384–389.

Pratt, B. L., & Goldman, B. D. (1986). Maternal influence on activity rhythms and reproductive development in Djungarian hamster pups. *Biology of Reproduction, 34*, 655–663.

Reppert, S. M. (1982). Maternal melatonin: a source of melatonin for the immature mammal. In D. C. Klein (Ed.), *Melatonin Rhythm Generating System* (pp, 182–191). Basel, Switzerland. S. Karger.

Reppert, S. M. (1987). Circadian rhythms: basic aspects and pediatric implications. In D. M. Styne (Ed.), *Current Concepts in Pediatric Endocrinology* (pp. 91–125). Holland. Elsevier.

Reppert, S. M., Chez, R. A., Anderson, A., & Klein, D. C. (1979). Maternal-fetal transfer of melatonin in a non-human primate. *Pediatric Research, 13*, 788–791.

Reppert, S. M., Coleman, R. J., Heath H. W., & Swedlow, J. R. (1984). Pineal N-acetyltransferase activity in 10-day-old rats: a paradigm for studying the developing circadian system. *Endocrinology, 115*, 918–925.

Reppert, S. M., Duncan, M. J., & Goldman, B. D. (1985). Photic influences on the developing mammal. *Ciba Foundation Symposium, 117*, 116–128.

Reppert, S. M., Henshaw, D., Schwartz, W. J., & Weaver, D. R. (1987). The circadian gated timing of birth in rats: disruption by maternal SCN lesions or by removal of the fetal brain. *Brain Research, 403*, 398–402.

Reppert, S. M., & Schwartz, W. J. (1983). Maternal coordination of the fetal biological clock in utero. *Science, 220*, 969–971.

Reppert, S. M., & Schwartz, W. J. (1984a). The suprachiasmatic nuclei of the fetal rat: characterization of a functional circadian clock using ^{14}C- labeled deoxyglucose. *Journal of Neuroscience, 4*, 1677–1682.

Reppert, S. M., & Schwartz, W. J. (1984b). Functional activity of the suprachiasmatic nuclei in the fetal primate. *Neuroscience Letters, 46*, 145–149.

Reppert, S. M., & Schwartz, W. J. (1986a). The maternal suprachiasmatic nuclei are necessary for maternal coordination of the developing circadian system. *Journal of Neuroscience, 6*, 2724–2729.

Reppert, S. M., & Schwartz, W. J. (1986b). Maternal endocrine extirpations do not abolish maternal coordination of the fetal circadian clock. *Endocrinology, 119*, 1763–1767.

Rivkees, S. A., Hall, D. A., Weaver, D. R., & Reppert, S. M. (1988). Djungarian hamsters exhibit reproductive responses to changes in day-length at extreme photoperiods. *Endocrinology 122*, 2634–2638.

Rossendale, P. D., & Short, R. V. (1967). The time of foaling of thoroughbred mares. *Journal of Reproduction and Fertility, 13*, 341–343.

Schwartz, W. J., Davidson, L. C., & Smith, C. B. (1980). In vivo metabolic activity of a putative circadian oscillator, the rat suprachiasmatic nucleus. *Journal of Comparative Neurology, 189*, 157–167.

Schwartz, W. J., & Gainer, H. (1977). Suprachiasmatic nucleus: Use of ^{14}C-labeled deoxyglucose uptake as a functional marker. *Science, 197*, 1089–1091.

Shibata, S., Liou, S. Y., & Ueki, S. (1983). Development of the circadian rhythm of neuronal activity in suprachiasmatic nucleus of rat hypothalamic slices. *Neuroscience Letters, 43* 231–234.

Sokoloff, L., Reivich, M., Kennedy, C., Des Rosiers, M. H., Patlak, C. S., Pettigrew, K. D., Sakurada, O., & Shinohara, M. (1977). *Journal of Neurochemistry, 28*, 897–916.

Stanfield, B., & Cowan, W. M. (1976). Evidence for a change in the retinohypothalamic projection in the rat following early removal of one eye. *Brain Research, 104*, 129–133.

Stephan, F. K. (1981). Limits of entrainment to periodic feeding in rats with suprachiasmatic lesions. *Journal of Comparative Physiology, 143*, 401–410.

Stetson, M. H., Elliott, J. A., & Goldman, B. D. (1986). Maternal transfer of photoperiodic information influences the photoperiodic response of prepubertal Djungarian hamsters (Phodopus sungorus sungorus). *Biology of Reproduction, 34,* 664–669.

Takahashi, J. S., DeCoursey, P. J., Bauman, L., & Menaker, M. (1984). Spectral sensitivity of a novel photoreceptive system mediating entrainment of mammalian circadian rhythms. *Nature, 308,* 186–188.

Takahashi, K., & Deguchi, T. (1983). Entrainment of the circadian rhythms of blinded infant rats by nursing mothers. *Physiology and Behavior, 31,* 373–378.

Tamarkin, L., Baird, C. J., & Almeida, O. F. X. (1985). Melatonin: A coordinating signal for mammalian reproduction? *Science, 227,* 714–720.

Tamarkin, L., Hollister, C. W., Lefebvre, N. G., & Goldman, B. D. (1977). Melatonin induction of gonadal quiescence in pinealectomized golden hamsters. *Science, 198,* 953–955.

Tamarkin, L., Reppert, S. M., Orloff, D. J., Klein, D. C., Yellon, S. M., & Goldman, B. D. (1980). Ontogeny of the pineal melatonin rhythm in the Syrian (*Mesocricetus auratus*) and Siberian (*Phodopus sungorus*) hamsters and in the rat. *Endocrinology, 107,* 1061–1064.

Viswanathan, N., & Chandrashekaran, M. K. (1984). Mother mouse sets the circadian clock of pups. *Proceedings of the Indian Academy of Sciences (Animals Science), 93,* 235–241.

Viswanathan, N., & Chandrashekaran, M. K. (1985). Cycles of presence and absence of mother mouse entrain the circadian clock of pups. *Nature, 317,* 530–531.

Weaver, D. R., & Reppert, S. M. (1986). Maternal melatonin communicates daylength to the fetus in Djungarian hamsters. *Endocrinology, 119,* 2861–2863.

Weaver, D. R., & Reppert, S. M. (1987). Maternal-fetal communication of circadian phase in a precocious rodent, the spiny mouse. *American Journal of Physiology, 253,* E401–E409.

Weaver, D. R., Keohan, J., & Reppert, S. M. (1987). Definition of a prenatal sensitive period for maternal-fetal communication of daylength. *American Journal of Physiology, 253,* E701–E704.

Weaver, D. R., Namboodiri, MAA, & Reppert, S. M. (1988). Iodinated melatonin mimics melatonin action and reveals discrete binding sites in fetal brain. *FEBS Letters 228,* 123–127.

Yellon, S. M., & Longo, L. D. (1987). Melatonin rhythms in fetal and maternal circulation during pregnancy in sheep. *American Journal of Physiology, 252,* E799–E802.

Yellon, S. M., Tamarkin, L., & Goldman, B. D. (1985). Maturation of the pineal melatonin rhythm in long– and short-day reared Djungarian hamsters. *Experientia, 41,* 651–652.

Zucker, I., Johnston, P. G., & Frost, D. (1980). Comparative, physiological and biochronometric analysis of rodent seasonal reproductive cycles. *Progress in Reproductive Biology, 5,* 102–133.

Environmental Stimulation and Human Fetal Responsivity in Late Pregnancy

Eugene K. Emory
Department of Psychology
Emory University
Atlanta, Georgia

Kay A. Toomey
Department of Psychology
State University of New York at Binghamton
Binghamton, New York

The human fetus remains something of an enigma, partly because it is often perceived as existing in a transitional state somewhere on the boundary between human and animal existence. It lives in a world more characteristic of aquatic mammals than human beings, and yet from these ontogenetically humble beginnings emerges an organism endowed with all the capacities for uniquely human functioning. It is perhaps fetal life, in comparison to all other stages of development, that marks our biological link to the animal kingdom. As a point of departure for psychobiological study, the human fetus and young infant offers the most advanced level of animal development and simultaneously the most primitive level of human existence. In this context, psychological theories about fetal development must provide novel conceptualizations which bridge the gap between animal and human development.

A major epoch in the study of fetal development commenced with the seminal volumes by Preyer (1888; 1889), which ushered in a new era of early ontogenetic study. In the 1920s, '30s, and '40s, several studies reported activity of the human fetus and began to document its responsivity to environmental stimulation (Forbes & Forbes, 1927; Peiper, 1925; Ray,

1932; Sontag & Wallace, 1934; Spelt, 1948). By far the most comprehensive and systematic study of the human fetus through 1971 was provided by Sontag (Sontag, 1941; 1971; Sontag & Wallace, 1934; 1935). With regard to contemporary issues of fetal responsivity and learning, two early studies deserve special note. They provided evidence, upon which many contemporary studies are based, that (a) during the last two months of pregnancy it is possible to establish a conditioned movement response in the human fetus that exhibits experimental extinction, spontaneous recovery, retention over a three week interval and high reliability between direct recording and maternal reports of fetal movement (Spelt, 1948), and (b) repeated external stimulation produces a progressive decrease in heart rate responsivity (Sontag, 1971). Therefore, for purpose of the current discussion, we emphasize that the potential for learning in the human fetus was seriously considered 40 years ago.

Many important contemporary issues focus upon methodology and are devoted to understanding the optimal conditions under which fetal learning takes place along with which response systems provide the most reliable evidence that such processes are operable. Theoretically, the question is how does the fetus process information and what are the psychobiological and cognitive mechanisms that account for this phenomenon?

Especially important for developmental psychobiology are questions about the nature of fetal responsivity to stressful experience during the perinatal, and especially parturitional, period. This is a particularly salient issue, because much of the stimulation to which the human fetus is exposed during the latter stages of labor is unquestionably stressful, emanating primarily from uterine activity. This stress not only requires adaptive physiological responses, but occasionally exhausts fetal reserves, leading to metabolic acidosis and fetal distress.

INDIVIDUAL DIFFERENCES

Consider the low risk situation in which labor is unremarkable and the fetus is delivered in a healthy state. Perhaps it is the healthy term fetus which responds in its own unique fashion that offer the greatest insights for developmental psychology. A recent literature suggests that individual differences among fetuses can be detected through observation of autonomic responses following stimulation. Welford and coworkers (1967) alluded to such a phenomenon when reporting the consistent individual patterns of sudden and dramatic drops in heart rate among fetal subjects. Converging evidence from temperament research (Coll, Resnick & Kagan, 1984; Kagan, Resnick, Clarke, Snidman & Garcia-Coll, 1984) suggests that unique individual temperamental styles are correlated with tonic heart rate during early childhood. Recently, Goldsmith and coworkers (1987) concluded that temperament is genetic in origin and appears in infancy. These traits are considered to provide the foundation for later personality. These and other anecdotal reports consistently reveal that if temperamental and rudimentary personality characteristics have biological correlates, they are most likely present during fetal life and may set the stage for reciprocal interactions between the perinate and its environment.

LEARNING AND COGNITION IN THE FETUS

Cardiac Orienting Response

A second major theme related to fetal development concerns the capacity for learning and cognition. What is now a considerable research literature began with the early work of Spelt (1948). The thrust of contemporary research related to learning and cognition in the human fetus dates back to earlier Soviet research on the orientating response (OR) and its cardiac components (Polinkamina & Probatova, 1965). This research, and subsequent studies in the U.S. (Adkinson & Berg, 1976; Berg, 1974; Graham & Clifton, 1966; Jackson, Kantowitz & Graham, 1971), documented that a cardiac component of the OR could be elicited in infants as young as six months of age. The cardiac response consists of a bradycardic episode following stimulus onset and then a return to baseline level. Berg (1974) helped to establish the lower age limit at which a heart rate deceleration to a novel non-aversive auditory signal could be elicited. Although at six weeks a heart rate deceleration could be elicited to an auditory signal, it was consistently more reliable at six months of age.

By implication, a failure to elicit cardiac orienting and habituation in very young infants (those under six weeks of age) and the increasing reliability with which the response can be observed as the infant grows older suggests that the young infant learns less or has a lower capacity for learning than the older child. This issue continued to perplex investigators studying human developmental psychophysiology. Kearsley (1973) reported that cardiac deceleration could be elicited in the newborn. The finding was not replicated for ten years, until Clarkson and Berg (1983) reported a reliable cardiac deceleration in 2–4 day old human neonates under very strict experimental conditions. They included the presentation of an auditory stimulus containing two important components: pulsed sounds with vowel like qualities. This finding has tremendous theoretical importance because it immediately links the conditions for eliciting a cardiac OR in the neonate to the ecological significance of certain types of sounds in the environment, namely, those produced by other human beings (see Fifer & Moon, this volume). Such a notion suggests that the newborn, and by extension the fetus, are genetically programmed to respond to certain auditory signals that enhance adaptation and increase survival.

Such findings leave unanswered the basic question of why the infant and neonate respond in the manner in which they do. Why is heart rate deceleration so difficult to elicit? In order to begin to answer such a question one must attempt to integrate the existing findings related to fetal and infant cardiac maturation. There appears to be more than one major factor involved in the development of the OR and its habituation.

There are at least two biological constraints that have not been investigated thoroughly. First, there is the constraint on cardiac function in the fetus and neonate that restricts the magnitude of cardiac deceleration in response to information from the environment. An infrequently discussed fact regarding cardiac function in the fetus and infant, which may help to clarify this issue, relates to the limited capacity to vary stroke volume when an increase in oxygen is needed. The characteristic of the fetal cardiovascular system that is important in this regard is high cardiac output, estimated to be approximately 200 ml/kg-min (Sandberg, 1978; Walsh & Lind, 1978). Cardiac output of this magnitude promotes fetal adaptation to the low oxygen tension of its blood in utero. Several studies have found that fetal cardiac muscles have limited variation in stroke volume when compared to an adult (Cohn, Piasecki & Jackson, 1978; Kirkpatrick & Freidman, 1978; Kirkpatrick, Naliboff, Pitbik & Freidman, 1975; Rudolph & Heyman, 1975). Thus the fetus operates to maximize its ability to provide sufficient oxygen. Therefore, the response of the fetus to an increased need for oxygenated blood is a significant rise in heart rate. With these biological constraints, it is understandably difficult to elicit a bradycardic episode in a healthy fetus in response to auditory stimulation. The same conclusions apply to the neonate and young infant. Maturation of the cardiac system is rapid during the first six months of life. Therefore, the infant is more capable of responding to novel auditory stimulation with a bradycardic episode because it is capable of varying its stroke volume and can maintain sufficiently oxygenated blood while simultaneously decreasing its heart rate.

A second constraint that has received recent attention is the maturation of the vagus nerve and its input to cardiac muscle. Early in gestation the fetal heart sets its own resting tone, with little variability. Some feel that during fetal and neonatal life, resting heart rate is maintained without significant autonomic influence, while changes are mediated through modification of intrinsic controlling mechanisms and changes in the action potential of myocardial cells (Freidman, 1973; Hopkins, McCutcheon & Weskstein, 1973). Assali and coworkers (1978) assert that in early gestation adrenergic tone is two to three times greater than cholinergic tone. During the third trimester, parasympathetic maturation approaches adult levels (Hon, Zannini & Quilligan, 1961). The increase in parasympathetic activity and maturation of the vagus are most likely simultaneous events. Vagal tone, which is activated in late gestation and early postnatal life, allows for the young organism to modulate its heart rate in response to stimulation (Porges et al., 1980). This parasympathetic activity not only enhances the organism's response to stimulation, but is responsible for beat-to-beat variability.

Vagal tone is thought to be related to the maturation of the central nervous system. Porges has developed an unbiased measure of vagal tone known as $\hat{V}$ (Larson, DiPietro & Porges, 1987; Porges, 1979) that controls for the association between heart rate and respiration (e.g., respiratory sinus arhythmia). Again, it is likely that the maturational process which leads to increased parasympathetic activity, coupled with the functional and anatomical changes in the cardiac muscle itself, sets the stage for the reliable elicitation of a heart rate deceleration in response to environmental stimulation. These constraints influence fetal and neonatal heart rate and prevent the organism from exhibiting the OR characteristic of the more mature individual.

A third constraint relates to the cognitive component of the orienting response itself. This constraint relates to what we might think of as cognition in the young infant. The OR is thought to enhance information processing on the part of the organism. It is a psychological phenomenon related to detection and registration of incoming stimulus information. If the organism is biologically capable, and also detects and registers the stimulus, then it is most likely to exhibit the cardiac deceleration component of the OR, which is thought to be a rudimentary component of early cognition and learning. But alone the OR, as represented by cardiac deceleration, does not imply learning. The learning component includes not only the "neuronal model" to which Sokolov (1975) has referred, but also to some aspect of stimulus selectivity. It is in this regard that another concept must be invoked to explain why the developing organism is more likely to demonstrate orienting and habituation as it gets older than the very immature fetus and neonate. Our hypothesis is that the young infant learns what information to attend to and what information is irrelevant. Speech sounds have ecological meaning and are capable under optimal conditions of eliciting an OR. However, other information in the environment does not carry with it such primordial significance and therefore

must be assimilated into the infant's early schema for processing information. What the young organism learns, therefore, is to pay attention to
certain information, which is secondary to the reflective orienting type
response.

As an example, the young infant may orient to almost any non-
threatening novel stimulation during the neonatal period. But very quickly
it learns that certain sounds in the environment have little consequence.
Therefore it does not respond with an OR to all stimuli. It learns for
example that certain stimuli which have unique characteristics may need
to be attended to. This conceptualization is basically a two-factor model
of cardiac orienting and habituation in the developing infant. It pre-
supposes that biological constraints, both cardiac and neuronal, restrict
the range of stimuli to which the organism can respond with heart rate
deceleration. Additionally, the need for the organism to not only detect
stimuli but to selectively process information provides the other condition
necessary for the OR. If and only if these conditions are met will one
observe complete expression of the cardiac orienting response and its
habituation.

Habituation

The issue of fetal habituation has been addressed more directly with
vibro-tactile stimulation. In two studies of fetal habituation, Leader and
coworkers (1982a; 1982b) induced movement by applying the base of an
electric toothbrush to the maternal abdomen, demonstrating that habituation occurred within 50 applications of the vibrating stimulus. They also
found that fetuses with CNS abnormalities did not respond to the vibrating
stimulus. In other high-risk fetuses there was a tendency toward responding, but habituation was accomplished more slowly than among normal
controls. Subsequently, Madison and coworkers (1986) demonstrated that
fetuses born at 40 weeks gestation not only habituated to repeated vibro-
tactile stimulation, but also dishabituated to the presentation of a novel
stimulus, habituated to the second stimulus, and showed a more rapid
response decrement to reapplication of the initial stimulus. The results of
these experiments clearly support the notion that fetal habituation can be
observed and measured reliably. Whether or not this effect can be demonstrated for the cardiovascular system remains to be determined.

There appears to be evidence for at least rudimentary forms of learning,
memory and cognition during the prenatal period. These findings have
direct implications for the neonatal work on the orienting response as

well as the usefulness of Porges's $\hat{V}$ or variability index. The notion that fetuses and young infants exhibit less reliable cardiac deceleration due to biological constraints can be tested directly by studying vibro-tactile and acoustic habituation in the same subject. A failure to find reliable heart rate deceleration to acoustic stimulation, but success in demonstrating habituation to vibro-tactile stimulation, would appear to support the biological constraint model. It will continue to be necessary to include a strong biological component in any theory of early development that includes the prenatal period.

An example of the close association between biology and psychology with respect to fetal and infant development is aptly demonstrated by the effects of clinical risk upon later behavioral development. It is well documented that severe prenatal insults and trauma can compromise psychological development. It is suggested here that the biological constraints placed upon the intact fetus parallel the influence of clincial risk upon the traumatized fetus. That is, normal development is more likely when biology is not adversely influenced, whereas biological insults and traumas compromise attainment of the individual's full potential. In this regard there will likely be social factors which also constrain the fetus but enhance the infant's capacity for orienting. The development of the cardiac orienting response and its habituation may well be imbedded in environmental factors and the social context.

CLINICAL ISSUES

Thus far, this essay has focused upon the healthy intact fetus and infant and devoted limited attention to the issues of clinical risk and developmental problems. This area is, however, at the forefront of controversy related to high-risk development and obstetric malpractice litigation. Much of high-risk infant research has been devoted to study of differences between normal full-term infants and their high-risk counterpart, be they premature or suffering from other clinical syndromes. What has emerged in the last twenty years is a resurgence of research on the fetus as it relates to clinical condition during gestation, labor and delivery. Much of this research has focused on describing the typography of the fetal cardiac response to uterine contractions during the latter stages of labor.

Early clinical studies of fetal heart rate (FHR) were from the Collaborative Perinatal Project, which concluded that FHR was not a reliable indicator of fetal distress (Benson, Shubeck, Deutschberger, Weiss, &

Berendes, 1968). Berendes (1969) found no differences in IQ scores at four years between children with low intrapartum FHR compared to those with normal FHR. Broman, Nicholes and Kennedy (1975) reported similar negative results. Schifrin and Dame (1972) have pointed out that over 50% of the FHR information is lost with auscultation. Moreover, fetal bradycardia alone is not a clinically ominous sign (Cibils, 1975; Freeman, 1974). Even so, Nelson and Ellenberg (1986) suggest severe fetal bradycardia predicts postnatal behavior.

Recent studies using continuous electronic fetal monitoring have generally found that neonatal behavior is related to FHR patterns. Scanlon, Suzuki, Shea and Tronick (1979) reported that fetuses with a positive Oxytocin[1] Challenge Test (OCT), which is based upon the occurrence of FHR decelerations, had a lower birthweight and ponderal index than a comparable group of fetuses with a negative OCT. The positive OCT group also obtained lower Brazelton scores (a test of newborn infant behavior; Brazelton, 1973) on items related to reflex performance and state organization. Recently, Emory, Walker and Cruz (1982) found that FHR accelerations predicted alertness and orientation scores on the Brazelton scale, while decelerations predicted physiological stability and arousal. In a one year follow-up of infants who exhibited FHR decelerations during labor, Painter, Depp and O'Donaghue (1978) found that abnormal fetal cardiac patterns (i.e., decelerations) were highly predictive (91%) of the number of abnormal neurological assessments obtained on a sample of 50 high-risk infants during the first year of life. Others have stated that the developmental problems noted by Painter and coworkers (1978) did not appear to have persisted into later childhood (Paneth & Stark, 1983).

Thus, the debate goes on. Unfortunately the controversy is frequently limited to one issue—whether a child is severely mentally retarded or has cerebral palsy—although psychologists are well aware that these two groups constitute a very small proportion of children identified with behavioral problems and learning disabilities. An important and largely ignored question is what role perinatal trauma and measures of fetal resilience, such as heart rate, play in the pathogenesis of less dramatic forms of developmental disability. Neonatal studies have reported atypical sleep patterns and non-optimal behavioral performance related to state and autonomic regulation among infants with FHR decelerations (Emory & Noonan, 1984a, 1984b; Emory, Noonan, & Porter, 1984). Dreier and Wolff (1972) found that term infants with a history of perinatal distress (50% had FHR decelerations) displayed diminished variability in non-nutritive sucking patterns, and greater variability in the duration of sucking burst than a comparable group of non-distressed newborns.

FETAL STRESS

A key factor in fetal research is not only the nature of the fetal response to stimulation but also the influence of stress upon fetal functioning, both short and long term. The birth process is a significant early stressor that involves a series of mechanical and chemical changes in the internal milieu of the fetus, demanding rapid adaptation. Cranial compression is often severe, which produces a dramatic shift in cardiopulmonary functioning (Yang, 1979). Labor, therefore, can be seen as constituting a series of recurrent stressors (contractions) with stress-free periods in between. Labor also satisfies the most stringent criteria for a stimulus-response contingency. A critical factor for meeting the adaptive demands of this situation is an intact CNS to help mediate appropriate levels of fetal oxygenation. If fetal resources are inadequate to meet these demands, the fetus may become distressed and experience hypoxia, tissue damage (especially within the CNS), and possibly intrapartum death (Mendez-Bauer, Arnt, Gulin, Escarcena & Caldeyro-Barcia, 1967; Prechtl, 1965). The fetus's adaptive physiological response to contractions determines its tolerance for stress, and is therefore an important indicator of fetal status (Hon et al., 1975). This adaptive physiological response is reflected in fetal heart rate patterns.

There are three major types of FHR patterning that are intricately tied to nervous system functioning and adaptation to the stressor: (a) baseline, consisting of the average FHR between periodic changes; (b) acceleration-periodic changes, consisting of transitory increases in FHR above baseline concomitant with uterine contractions; and (c) deceleration-periodic changes, consisting of transitory decreases in FHR below baseline occurring with contractions. Variations within these three types of patterning during the last hour of labor are indicative of fetal status. Typically, the FHR response in the last 60 minutes of labor is studied because the most significant differences between compromised and uncompromised perinates are observed at this time (Cibils, 1975; Emory et al., 1982). Generally a fetus exhibits one of three global patterns of FHR response during this time period (Figure 1): (a) FHR accelerations in response to contractions, (b) FHR decelerations with contractions, or (c) initial heart rate accelerations followed by decelerations just prior to delivery. Mendez-Bauer and coworkers (1963) demonstrated that there are two components to the decelerations: vagal tone and direct hypoxia of the myocardium. Cranial hypertension or stimulation of the brain develops from uterine compression and results in stimulation of the vagus center. This increased vagal tone in turn results in FHR deceleration. This pattern can be blocked by atropine, a parasympathetic inhibitor, thereby supporting the

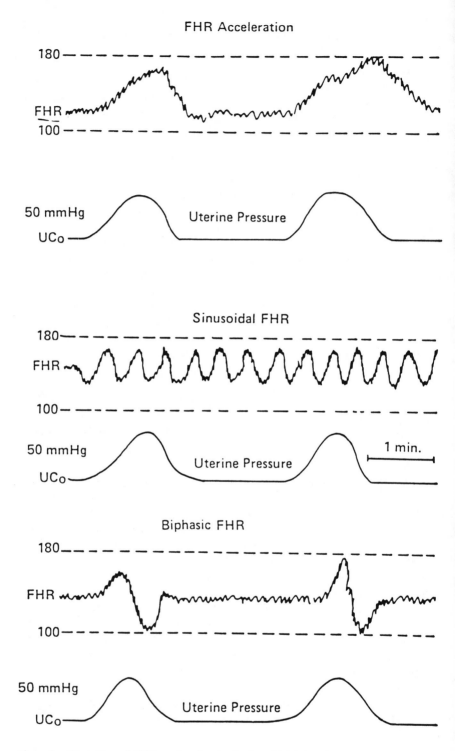

Figure 1. Illustration of FHR acceleration (top), sinusoidal (middle), and biphasic (bottom) patterns of response.

primary role of vagal tone (Mendez-Bauer et al., 1963). This type of pattern is associated with head compression (Figure 2, top). The relationship between this manifestation of vagal tone and Porge's $\hat{V}$ have not been determined. The late deceleration pattern (Figure 2, middle) is the result of more complex processes (Table 1).

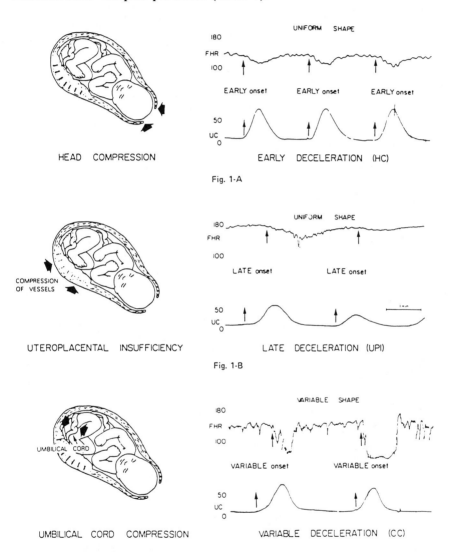

HEAD COMPRESSION   EARLY DECELERATION (HC)

Fig. 1-A

UTEROPLACENTAL INSUFFICIENCY   LATE DECELERATION (UPI)

Fig. 1-B

UMBILICAL CORD COMPRESSION   VARIABLE DECELERATION (CC)

Figure 2. Illustration of the three most commonly observed FHR deceleration patterns. (adapted from Hon, et al., 1975).

Table 1: MODEL OF FHR DECELERATIONS

(MODIFIED FROM MENDEZ-BAUER, ET AL., 1963)

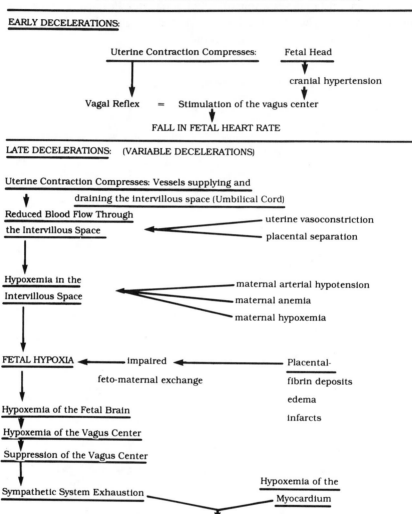

EARLY DECELERATIONS:

Uterine Contraction Compresses: Fetal Head

cranial hypertension

Vagal Reflex   =   Stimulation of the vagus center

FALL IN FETAL HEART RATE

LATE DECELERATIONS: (VARIABLE DECELERATIONS)

Uterine Contraction Compresses: Vessels supplying and
draining the intervillous space (Umbilical Cord)

Reduced Blood Flow Through
the Intervillous Space   uterine vasoconstriction
                                          placental separation

Hypoxemia in the
Intervillous Space   maternal arterial hypotension
                                          maternal anemia
                                          maternal hypoxemia

FETAL HYPOXIA   impaired   Placental-
                 feto-maternal exchange   fibrin deposits
                                          edema
Hypoxemia of the Fetal Brain   infarcts

Hypoxemia of the Vagus Center

Suppression of the Vagus Center

                                          Hypoxemia of the
Sympathetic System Exhaustion   Myocardium

FALL IN FETAL HEART RATE

Normally, each uterine contraction causes a transient fall in fetal partial oxygen pressure (pO_2). A well oxygenated fetus may accelerate in response to this fall, or may show early decelerations if fetal head compression is occurring. However, if a compromising pre— or perinatal condition, such as uteroplacental insufficiency or intramyometrial vessel compression already exists, the fetal O_2 level cannot be fully recovered after each contraction. These conditions cause reduced blood flow through the intervillous space, thereby reducing the available O_2. The cumulative effect of these repeated events, as caused by each contraction, is that metabolic and respiratory acidosis develop and lead to hypoxia (Kunzel, Mann, Bhakthavathsalan, & Ayromlooi, 1978; Mendez-Bauer et al., 1963). Hypoxia of the brain disrupts vagus control first. This suppression of vagal tone releases the sympathetic system from inhibition, and a concomitant rise in heart rate baseline (tachycardia), along with lowered baseline variability, occurs. This is why tachycardia is the first sign that fetal O_2 debt is being compensated by an increase in heart rate. Results of experiments with propranolol, a sympathetic blocking drug, support sympathetic control of this process (Renou, Newman and Wood, 1969).

As hypoxia continues, the sympathetic system becomes severely compromised and hypoxia of the myocardium also develops. When this coincides with a contraction, depleted oxygen stores fall below a critical level, transient augmentation of vagal tone takes place, and a precipitous drop in FHR occurs (Kunzel et al., 1978; Pose, Castillo, Mora-Rojas, Soto-Yances & Caldeyro-Barcia, 1969). Caldeyro-Barcia and coworkers (1973) hypothesized that one uterine contraction can cause a late deceleration when that contraction also produces a fall in O_2 below a critical level. Indeed, Bieniarz and coworkers (1965) found that late decelerations occurred when maternal hypotension depleted fetal reserves below a critical level. Current neurological studies using PET scans have found that as compensatory mechanisms for oxygen extraction become exhausted, oxygen metabolism falls as it reaches a critical utilization rate. At this point the percentage of O_2 extracted by the cerebral tissue also declines (Phelps & Mazziotta, 1985). The late onset of the deceleration is due, then, to the time lapse between contraction peak and O_2 depletion to the critical point. That the late decelerations can be reduced or abolished by raising fetal pO_2 supports oxygen status as the key variable of the pattern production (Caldeyro-Barcia et al., 1973; James et al., 1972). As the contraction releases, thereby increasing circulation, the exhausted sympathetic system slowly returns the FHR to a now lowered overall baseline. If hypoxia continues to worsen, the situation approaches total exhaustion of metabolic reserves, and asphyxia and fetal death may result.

Umbilical cord compression allows for a situation of intermittent full doses of O_2 to be received by the fetus, and produces the variable deceleration patterns shown in Figure 2 (bottom). This pattern becomes progressively worse as the drops increase in frequency and duration (Hon et al., 1975). It takes longer in this intermittent O_2 situation for the oxygen levels to become depleted to exhaustion and to fall below the critical level. Again, if the hypoxic events continue to recur, the situation may become severe enough to approach the circumstance of asphyxia (see Figure 2).

GLOBAL FHR PATTERNS

We have found that there are significant differences in perinatal outcome in fetuses that demonstrate a pattern of FHR acceleration throughout the last hour of labor compared to those that show a consistent deceleration or pattern of mixed acceleration and deceleration. Whereas fetuses that exhibit consistently accelerated heart rate during delivery have good Apgar scores at birth and few perinatal problems, fetuses that demonstrate a pattern of deceleration have lower birthweights, more perinatal problems, and lower scores on neonatal assessments (Cibils, 1975; Emory & Noonan, 1984a; 1984b; Powell, Melville & Mackenna, 1979). These latter fetuses have poorer developmental outcomes up to one year of age (Painter et al., 1978). The fetuses showing the mixed pattern of FHR acceleration and deceleration have developmental outcomes at four months of age that are generally superior to the other two groups (Toomey, Emory, & Savoie, 1987). This is a surprising finding, given that deceleration has been hypothesized as being indicative of hypoxia in myocardial and, possibly, brain tissue. One would expect this mixed FHR response group to perform intermediate to the other groups on developmental measures. The explanation for the superior performance of the mixed group may be found in Selye's model of stress (Selye, 1936; 1979), known as the General Adaptation Syndrome (GAS).

Selye (1980, p. vii) defines stress as "the nonspecific (that is common) result of *any* demand upon the body, be it a mental or somatic demand, for survival...." Biological stress is specifically seen to be linked to utilization of energy reserves. The GAS model outlines a tripartite physiological-behavioral response to any stressor: an alarm reaction, a stage of resistance, and finally exhaustion. The alarm reaction consists of two phases that occur when an organism is exposed to a noxious, nonadapted stimulus. The organism's initial and immediate response to the stressor is labelled as the "shock" phase. Then a rebound "countershock" phase occurs in which the organism's defense mechanisms are mobilized. If the stressor continues, the organism will enter a stage of resistance in which symptoms are generally alleviated and full adaptation to the stressor occurs. However, should the stressor continue beyond the organism's finite level of "adaptation energy", exhaustion will occur. There are two types of adaptation energy: one which is easily available, but also superficial and easily depleted, and another that is more slowly mobilized, but is more deep-seated and extensive. The exhaustion phase is characterized by local tissue necrosis and premature death if the stressors are severe enough. Table 2 outlines a conceptual formulation of the type of FHR response as it parallels Selye's GAS model.

The stressor in this conceptualization is the uterine contraction. Changes in FHR in response to this stressor reflect the stages of the fetus's ongoing adaptation. The exact pattern of change that occurs depends on the individual fetus's conditioning factors, a combination of pre-existing conditions and genetic predispositions. The alarm reaction consists of a periodic change with each contraction. The shock phase involves the initial change in FHR from baseline (acceleration of deceleration), and the countershock phase begins at the point of maximum amplitude deviation. The stage of resistance consists of the return to baseline. Lastly, the exhaustion phase is characterized by severe and repetitive variable or late deceleration, with a loss of heart rate variability.

In our conceptualization, fetuses that exhibit FHR acceleration during contraction have good metabolic reserves at the onset of labor. That is, they have a large store of the first of the two "adaptation energy" levels discussed by Selye (1976). Although they do tap into the second level of adaptation energy, their catecholamine mobilization is not strong. Conversely, fetuses that respond with FHR deceleration have depleted reserves

Table 2

Hypothesized Relationship between Stages of
the General Adaptation Syndrome and Fetal Heart Response

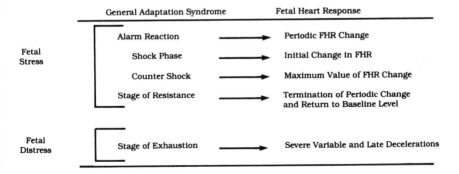

	General Adaptation Syndrome	Fetal Heart Response
Fetal Stress	Alarm Reaction	Periodic FHR Change
	Shock Phase	Initial Change in FHR
	Counter Shock	Maximum Value of FHR Change
	Stage of Resistance	Termination of Periodic Change and Return to Baseline Level
Fetal Distress	Stage of Exhaustion	Severe Variable and Late Decelerations

of oxygen and the first level of adaptation energy. They move rapidly toward exhaustion of the second level of adaptation energy, and their catecholamine response is exceptionally large. The fetuses that exhibit a mixed acceleration-deceleration response begin with adequate reserves of the first level of adaptation energy. At some point in labor, probably due to unique predispositions, these reserves are depleted and there is a shift to utilization of the second level of adaptation energy, coupled with a moderate amount of catecholamine mobilization.

Why are catecholamines so critical in the FHR-GAS conceptualization? First, catecholamines may be directly related to Selye's second adaptation energy level. Second, catecholamines are a critical component of fetal status during labor and delivery. Lagercrantz and Slotkin (1986) found that when a human fetus is deprived of oxygen, the adrenal glands release catecholamines into plasma. At this point, the hypoxic or anoxic condition approaches exhaustion, as proposed by Selye (1979). In addition, Lagercrantz and Slotkin assert that catecholamines, specifically NE, elicit a reflexive slowing of heart rate which is mediated by the vagus. The reduction promotes fetal survival by decreasing the heart's oxygen needs, and by reducing the stress on the heart due to an accelerated operational level. This response is similar to that in diving marine animals; the dive causes catecholamine levels to rise, peripheral blood flow to decrease, blood to be redirected to the vital organs, and heart rate to slow. Lagercrantz and Slotkin state that a catecholamine surge is necessary for a fetus or newborn to survive hypoxia. What is likely to be observed in the clinical situation is an early deceleration.

Given that catecholamine surges and concomitant FHR deceleration, mediated by the vagus, serve a protective function, one may expect that fetuses demonstrating early bradycardia would be more vigorous at birth. This is exactly the finding of Lagercrantz and Slotkin (1986). Infants that were delivered by planned cesarian section had low catecholamine levels at birth, vaginally delivered infants had moderate levels, and asphyxiated infants had extraordinarily high levels. Vaginally delivered newborns with moderate levels of catecholamines had better lung compliance shortly after birth, enhanced blood flow to vital organs, immediate mobilization of metabolites for energy, and were more alert than newborns in the other two groups. Catecholamine surges facilitate normal breathing in newborns, and sustained catecholamine increases in the hours prior to delivery are important for adequate surfactant release and adsorption of lung fluids after birth (Lagercrantz & Slotkin, 1986). This effect in new-borns is particularly adaptive as there is no longer a continual stream of nutrients flowing from the placenta. Infants with low catecholamine levels are said to often have low blood sugar levels as well. Infants with moderate catecholamine levels also appear more alert and have dilated pupils immediately after birth. This particular effect has been suggested to facilitate maternal-infant bonding (Lagercrantz & Slotkin, 1986).

In summary, fetuses that show FHR acceleration during labor are hypothesized to have good pre-existing metabolic reserves, so they do not experience a complete shift to utilization of the second level of adaptation energy. These babies, upon delivery, are similar to the surgically delivered infants in the Lagercrantz and Slotkin study. They are not compromised, but neither do they benefit from catecholamine effects. One should expect these newborns to perform fairly well on measures that tap exploratory and approach responses, given their corticoid exposure as an initial result of stress.

Fetuses that exhibit the mixed FHR pattern begin with adequate reserves of the first energy level for responding to stress, as reflected in the initial FHR acceleration. However, with depletion of this reserve a shift to the second energy level occurs. Moderate catecholamine mobilization results in catecholamine surges and concomitant decelerations. This results in a superior neonatal condition that continues to be exhibited on developmental indices.

Fetuses that exhibit FHR deceleration have virtually no reserves of the first energy level, due to some compromising pre-existent condition. These fetuses enter the last hour of labor far into the second level of energy reserves; catecholamine mobilization is rapid and excessive. As the hypoxic conditions continue, oxygen as well as energy reserves are depleted. The compensatory mechanisms usually initiated by catecholamine mobilization begin to fail, and the critical oxygen utilization rate is exceeded. The constant, high levels of catecholamines observed under these conditions may be indicative of the disruption in vagal control (Table 1). It appears that this group of neonates do not benefit from the effects generally observed with catecholamine mobilization; the positively influencing effects are negated by disruptive levels of catecholamines.

CONCLUDING REMARKS

Fetal life comprises many dynamics that have relevance for developmental psychobiology as well as general human development. Space limitations have not permitted a full discussion of other aspects of fetal life, including fetal breathing movements, general body movements in response to stimulation, and particular interactions between the fetus and mother that facilitate early infant-parent interaction. What has been discussed in some detail are the biological and psychological factors that place the fetus in a unique position, both ontogenetically and physiologically. Whether rudimentary temperament, personality, and individual differences are evident in fetal responses needs further investigation. The body of literature presented clearly supports the notion that genetic or constitutional factors probably exist prenatally and set the stage for early interactions that shape the course of future experience. Indeed, fetal research may have direct implications for risk research in psychopathology (Emory, Mapp, Hudgman, & Walker, 1984).

We have also suggested that biological constraints play an important role in the development of learning and cognition. These constraints are perhaps most unique in the fetus, with a cardiovascular system that is undergoing rapid change. Change also extends into the neonatal period, where maturation of myocardial fibers continues during the first year of life. It is in this context that explanations regarding the origin and development of the cardiac component of the orienting response become meaningful. Of particular importance is the potential for predicting the onset of the cardiac component of the orienting response and its habituation over time. Linking these concepts together promotes the view that early evaluation and prediction of learning and cognitive function becomes possible as methodology continues to be refined.

Finally, we have discussed stress responses and the mediating effects of catecholamine surges during the latter stages of labor. These are biochemical phenomena that seem to be directly related to the capacity of the organism to respond to subsequent stimulation. Although counterintuitive, the discussion concludes that a fetus, stressed moderately by labor, which can mobilize its energy reserves, is likely to respond in a superior manner over other fetuses during the early neonatal period. This type of response is analogous to stress inoculation, whereby the fetus that is moderately stressed, but not overly compromised, receives the greatest benefit from the process of labor. As these examples of recent research illustrate, the area of fetal development offers unlimited opportunities for ontogenetic study and promises to be one of the most exciting endeavors in human psychological research.

Acknowledgements

Preparation of the chapter was supported by National Science foundation Grant #BSN-8696151 to the first author.

References

Adkinson, C. D., & Berg, W. K. (1976). Cardiac deceleration in newborns: habituation, dishabituation and offset responses. *Journal of Experimental Child Psychology*, *21*, 46–60.

Assali, N. S., Brinkman, C. R., Woods, R., Jr., Dandavino, A., & Nuwayhid, B. (1978). Ontogenesis of the autonomic control of cardiovascular function in the sheep. In L. Longo & D. Reneau, (Eds.), *Fetal and newborn cardiovascular physiology*, (vol. 1). New York: Garland STPM Press.

Benson, R. C., Shubeck, F., Deutschberger, J., Weiss, W., & Berendes, H. (1968). Fetal heart rate as a predictor of fetal distress. *American Journal of Obstetrics and Gynecology*, *32*, 259–266.

Berendes, H. W. (1969). Fetal distress: its significance in neurological and mental impairment of childhood. In Perinatal factors affecting human development. No. 185. Washington, D. C.: Pan American Health Organization.

Berg, W. K. (1974). Cardiac orienting responses of 6- and 16-week-old infants. *Journal of Experimental Child Psychology*, *17*, 303–312.

Bieniarz, J., Feranandez-Sepulveda, R., & Caldeyro-Barcia, R. (1965). Effects of maternal hypotension on the human fetus. *American Journal of Obstetrics and Gynecology*, *92*, 821-831.

Brazelton, T. B. (1973). Neonatal behavior assessment scale. *Clinics in developmental medicine, no. 50*. Philadelphia: Lippincott.

Broman, S. H., Nicholes, P. J., & Kennedy, N. (1975). *Preschool IQ: prenatal and early developmental correlates*. Hillsdale, NJ: Erlbaum.

Caldeyro-Barcia, R., Mendez-Bauer, C., Pose, S., & Poseiro, J. J. (1973). Fetal monitoring in labor. In H. Wallace, E. M. Gold, & E. F. Lis, (Eds.), *Maternal and child health practices*. Springfield, IL: Charles Thomas Publishers.

Cibils, L. (1975). Clinical significance of fetal heart rate patterns during labor. II. Late decelerations. *American Journal of Obstetrics and Gynecology*, *123*, 473–494.

Clarkson, M. G., & Berg, W. K. (1983). Cardiac orienting and vowel discrimination in newborns: crucial stimulus parameters. *Child Development*, *54*, 162–171.

Cohn, H., Piasecki, G. J., & Jackson, B. T. (1978). The role of autonomic nervous control in the fetal cardiovascular response to hypoxemia. In L. Longo & D. Reneau, (Eds.), *Fetal and newborn cardiovascular physiology*, (vol. 2). New York: Garland STPM Press.

Coll, C. G., Resnick, J., & Kagan, J. (1984). Behavioral inhibition in young children. *Child Development*, *55*, 1001–1019.

Dreier, T., & Wolff, P. (1972). Sucking, state, and perinatal distress in newborns. *Biology of the Neonate*, *21*, 16–24.

Emory, E. K. Mapp, J. R., Hodgman, J., & Walker, E. F. (1984). Approaches to high-risk research. *Biological Psychiatry*, *4*, 637–641.

Emory, E. K., & Noonan, J. R. (1984a). Fetal cardiac responding: maturational and behavioral correlates. *Developmental Psychology*, *20*, 354–357.

Emory, E. K., & Noonan, J. R. (1984b). Fetal cardiac responding: a predictor of birthweight and neonatal behavioral performance. *Child Development*, *55*, 651–657.

Emory, E. K. Noonan, J. R., & Porter, L. (1984). Behavioral implications of fetal cardiac responding. *International Journal of Psychophysiology*, *1*, 113–114.

Emory, E. K., Walker, E., & Cruz, A. (1982). Fetal heart rate part II: behavior correlates. *Psychophysiology*, *19*, 680–686.

Forbes, H. S., & Forbes, H. B. (1927). Fetal sense reactions: hearing. *Journal of Comparative Psychology*, *7*, 353–355.

Freeman, R. (1974). Intrapartum fetal evaluation. *Clinical Obstetrics and Gynecology*, *17*, 83–94.

Freidman, W. F. (1973). The intrinsic physiologic properties of the developing heart. In W. F. Freidman, M. Leach, & E. H. Sonnenblick, (Eds.), *Neonatal heart disease*. New York: Grune & Stratton.

Goldsmith, H. H., Buss, A. H., Plomin, R., Rothbart, M. K., Thomas, A., Chess, S., Hinde, R. A., & McCall, R. B. (1987). Roundtable: what is temperament? Four approaches. *Child Development*, *58*, 505–529.

Graham, F. K., & Clifton, R. K. (1966). Heart-rate changes as a component of the orienting response. *Psychological Bulletin*, *65*, 305–320.

Hon, E. H., Zannini, D., & Quilligan, E. J. (1975). The neonatal value of fetal monitoring. *American Journal of Obstetrics and Gynecology*, *122*, 508–519.

Hopkins, S. F., McCutcheon, E. P., & Weskstein, D. R. (1973). Postnatal changes in ventricular function. *Circulation Research*, *32*, 685–691.

Jackson, J. C., Kantowitz, S. R., & Graham, F. K. (1971). Can newborns show cardiac orienting? *Child Development*, *42*, 107–121.

James, L. S., Morishima, H., Daniel, S., Bowe, E., Cohen, H., & Neiman, W. (1972). Mechanism of late deceleration of the fetal heart rate. *American Journal of Obstetrics and Gynecology*, *113*, 578–582.

Kagan, J., Resnick, J. S., Clarke, C., Snidman, N., & Garcia-Coll, C. (1984). Behavioral inhibition to the unfamiliar. *Child Development*, *55*, 2212–2225.

Kearsley, R. B. (1973). The newborn's response to auditory stimulation: A demonstration of orienting and defensive behavior. *Child Development*, *44*, 582–590.

Kirkpatrick, S. E., & Freidman, W. F. (1978). Myocardial determinants of fetal cardiac output. In L. Longo & D. Reneau, (Eds.), *Fetal and newborn cardiovascular physiology*, (vol. 1). New York: Garland STPM Press.

Kirkpatrick, S. E., Naliboff, J., Pitbik, P. T., & Freidman, W. F. (1975). The influence of post stimulation potentiation and heart rate on the fetal lamb heart. *American Journal of Physiology*, *229*, 318–323.

Kunzel, W., Mann, L. I., Bhakthavathsalan, A., & Ayromlooi, J. (1978). Metabolic fetal brain function and cardiovascular observations following total cord occlusion. In L. D. Longo & D. D. Reneau, (Eds.), *Fetal and newborn cardiovascular physiology*, (vol. 2). New York: Garland STPM Press.

Lagercrantz, H., & Slotkin, T. A. (1986). The "stress" of being born. *Scientific American*, *254*, 100–107.

Larson, S. K., DiPietro, J. A., & Porges, S. W. (1987). Neonatal V and NBAS performance are related to developmental course at 15 months. Paper presented at Biennial Meeting of Society for Research in Child Development.

Leader, L. R., Baillie, P., Martin, b., & Vermuelen, E. (1982a). Fetal habituation in high-risk pregnancies. *British journal of Obstetrics and Gynecology*, *89*, 441–446.

Leader, L. R., Baillie, P., Martin, B., & Vermuelen, E. (1982b). The assessment and significance of habituation to a repeated stimulus by the human fetus. *Early Human Development*, *7*, 211–219.

Madison, L. S., Adubato, S. A., Madison, J. K., Nelson, R. B., Anderson, R., Erickson, J., Kuss, L., & Goodlin, R. C. (1986). Fetal response decrement: True habituation? *Journal of Developmental and Behavioral Pediatrics*, *7*, 14–20.

Mendez-Bauer, C., Arnt, I. C., Gulin, L. Escarcena, L., & Caldeyro-Barcia, R. (1967). Relationship between blood pH and heart rate in the human fetus during labor. *American Journal of Obstetrics and Gynecology*, *97*, 530–545.

Mendez-Bauer, C., Poseiro, J. J., Arellano-Hernandez, G., Zambrana, M. A., & Caldeyro-Barcia, R. (1963). Effects of atropine on the heart rate of the human fetus during labor. *American Journal of Obstetrics and Gynecology*, *85*, 1033–1053.

Nelson, K. B., & Ellenberg, J. H. (1986). Antecedents of cerebral palsy. Multivariate analysis of risk. *New England Journal of Medicine*, *315*, 81–86.

Painter, M. J., Depp, R., & O'Donaghue, P. D. (1978). Fetal heart rate patterns and development in the first year of life. *American Journal of Obstetrics and Gynecology*, *132*, 271–276.

Paneth, N., & Stark, R. I. (1983). Cerebral palsy and mental retardation in relation to indicators of perinatal asphyxia. *American Journal of Obstetrics and Gynecology*, *147*, 960.

Peiper, A. (1925). Sinnesempfindungen des Kindes vor seiner Geburt. *Monatsschrift fur Kinderheihkunde*, *29*, 236–241.

Sokolov, E. N. (1975). The neuronal mechanisms of the orienting reflex. In E. N. Sokolov & O. S. Vinogradova, (Eds.), *Neuronal mechanisms of the orienting reflex*, (pp. 217–235). Hillsdale, NJ: Lawrence Erlbaum Associates.

Sontag, L. W. (1941). The significance of fetal environmental differences. *American Journal of Obstetrics and Gynecology*, *42*, 996–1003.

Sontag, L. W. (1971). The history of longitudinal research: implications for the future. *Child Development*, *42*, 987–1000.

Sontag, L. W., & Wallace, R. F. (1934). Preliminary report of the Fels Fund, study of fetal activity. *American Journal of Diseases of Children*, *48*, 1050–1057.

Sontag, L. W., & Wallace, R. F. (1935). The movement response of the human fetus to sound stimuli. *Child Development*, *6*, 353–358.

Spelt, D. (1948). The conditioning of the human fetus in utero. *Journal of Experimental Psychology*, *51*, 583–589.

Toomey, K., Emory, E. K., & Savoie, T. (1987). Prediction from intrapartum fetal heart rate to four month infant development. Paper presented at Biennial Meeting for Society for Reseach in Child Development.

Walsh, S. Z., & Lind, J. (1978). The fetal circulation and its alteration at birth. In U. Stave, (Ed.), *Perinatal physiology*. New York: Plenum Medical.

Welford, N. T., Sontag, L. W., Phillips, W., & Phillips, D. (1967). Individual differences in heart rate variability in the human fetus. *American Journal of Obstetrics and Gynecology*, *98*, 56–61.

Yang, R. K. (1979). Early assessment: an overview. In J. Osofsky, (Ed.), *Handbook of infant development*, (pp. 165–184). New York: John Wiley and Sons.

Morphological consequences of depressed or impaired fetal activity

Adrien C. Moessinger
Department of Pediatrics
College of Physicians and Surgeons
Columbia University
New York, New York

"Dans tout animal qui n'a point depasse le terme de ses developments, l'emploi plus frequent et soutenu d'un organe... le developpe, l'agrandit et lui donne une puissance proportionnee a la duree de cet emploi; tandis que le defaut constant d'usage de cet organe l'affaiblit insensiblement, le deteriore, diminue progressivement ses facultes,...."

Lamark, *Philosophie Zoologique*, Paris 1809

There is mounting evidence derived both from scrutiny of "experiments of nature" in the human species and from experiments conducted with animal models to support the concept that function is an integral part of structural development during prenatal ontogeny. The available data specifically suggest that movement produced by muscular activity is an important determinant of normal morphological development. Most of the evidence for this conclusion is inferred from cases in which fetal activity is reduced or absent, because hypoactivity is more readily identified and induced than hyperactivity. This essay, therefore, will focus on situations where fetal movement is either intrinsically depressed (such as results from fetal myoneuropathy) or impaired by extrinsic constraint (such as may be produced by a malformed uterus). The morphological consequences of such hypokinesia or akinesia thus provide an important source of inference about the importance of normal fetal activity for the development of the fetus.

PHYSICAL FORCES AND MORPHOGENESIS

Although the ill effects of fetal immobility or constraint have been documented in several organ systems (muscles and skeleton, skin, gut,

163

lungs), congenital limb deformities have historically attracted the most attention. Hippocrates considered the malformation of limbs and believed that mechanical molding of the fetus in utero was a significant etiological factor. He compared the growing limbs of a fetus to the roots of a tree which, when hindered by a stone or other object, are bent during growth. Nicolas Andry further developed this analogy when he wrote his treatise entitled "Orthopaedics" (the art of straightening children) in 1741. Andry was particularly concerned with the treatment of crooked legs: "In a word, the same method must be used in this case, for recovering the shape of a leg, as is used for making straight the crooked trunc of a young tree." Andry's tree is the modern international symbol of orthopedic surgery.

There are indeed several points of similarity that can be identified when comparing the structure and growth of trees and bones. The collagen fibrils and the trabecules within the bone correspond to the cellulose fibers of a tree; because both become aligned in the direction of mechanical stress, the deforming effects of tensile, compressive and shear forces (angular distortion) are minimized. The role of mechanical forces in morphogenesis, and the means by which nature solves complex bioengineering problems by structural design, was the subject of D'Arcy W. Thompson's classic work, *On Growth and Form* (1942). More recently, Thompson's erudite work has been simply and succinctly recast in a beautifully illustrated chapter by David Smith (1981). Smith has elaborated on Thompson's observations with new hypotheses that shed light on the pathogenesis of several "malformation patterns". In fact, a substantial group of malformations are actually deformations which arise not from embryonic errors in morphogenesis, but rather are acquired in utero through alteration in the form or structure of an organ that retains full potential for normal growth but is subjected to abnormal biomechanical forces (Dunn, 1976). There are numerous examples in nature of the impact of physical forces, including mechanical, osmotic and electromagnetic forces, on morphogenesis (Thompson, 1942). For the sake of simplicity, the discussion below will focus on the role of mechanical forces in abnormal fetal development.

Mechanical forces can arise from one of two general sources: intrinsic to the growing organism, or extrinsic, imposed on the organism from its external environment. Intrinsic forces are generated by growth itself, such as by cell multiplication and hypertrophy. The action of intrinsic mechanical forces is evident in the development of contiguous organs, which are shaped by three dimensional restraint and the mechanical characteristics of the cytoskeleton. The shape of the liver, for instance, is quite different when it grows in an abnormal location, such as is seen with omphaloceles (congenital herniation into the umbilical cord), where the liver is molded to conform to a new set of contiguous structures. The abnormal development of an organ or growth of a tumor will exert similar forces that act on neighboring organs or surrounding tissues. Such an effect is evident in the growth of the skull and scalp in cases of hydrocephaly (an excessive accumulation of fluid within or surrounding the brain).

Muscle contraction obviously can exert mechanical force on the skeleton and joints, but muscle activity also has an impact on the entire cardiovascular system (from the pulsatile flow generated by the myocardium), the gut (from swallowing and peristalsis), and the lungs (from fetal breathing movements). The skin surrounding joints also is subjected to stretch and relaxation during motor activity and movement of joints. Intrinsic mechanical forces also are generated by alterations in the fluid balance within organs. Changes in the relative rates of secretion and excretion or resorption of body fluids affects the growth of the brain (in the ventricular system), the urinary and gastrointestinal tracts, and the fetal lungs. In summary, intrinsic forces are generated by (a) growth of organs and fetal mass, (b) muscle contractions by the fetus, and (c) changes in the flow or volume of body fluids.

Mechanical forces arising from extrinsic sources can act either directly, by exerting pressure or inducing stretch on a part of the fetus, or indirectly, by interfering with the normal expression of intrinsic forces. Direct effects are evident in instances where the intrauterine space is abnormal, such as in cases of unicornuate uterus, large fibromas (tumors of fibrous connective tissue), or oligohydramnios (reduced volume of amniotic fluid). Indirect action of extrinsic force can result from external restriction of the range of movement, thereby limiting the kinds and amounts of movement that can be performed by the fetus. The most common sources of extrinsic force during fetal development are (a) physical restraint within the uterus, (b) external compression, and (c) effects of gravity.

FETAL AKINESIA DEFORMATION SEQUENCE

It will be useful at this point to review the definition of some terms that are used in reference to specific examples of dysmorphology related to depressed or impaired fetal activity (Spranger, et al., 1982). "Malformation" is used when the defective formation of a tissue results from an intrinsically abnormal developmental process (e.g., renal agenesis, the complete absence of one or both kidneys). A "deformation" is an abnormal form, shape, or position of a part of the body caused by extrinsic mechanical forces (e.g., club foot induced by fetal restraint). "Disruption" denotes an extrinsic force that results in the breakdown of a previously normal tissue (e.g., limb amputation resulting from amniotic bands). Because

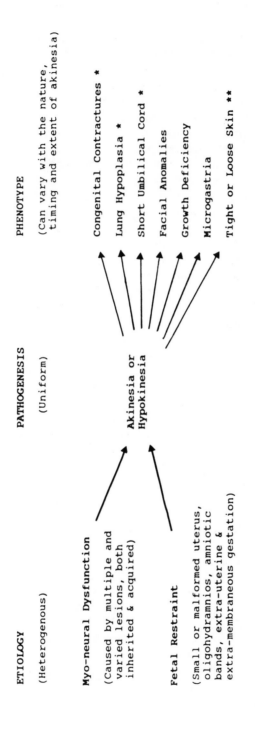

Figure 1. The Fetal Akinesia/Hypokinesia Deformation Sequence.

* Can lead to perinatal asphyxia and thus compound the neurological status.

** The skin tends to be tight and thin with myo-neural dysfunction and loose with abundant folds in cases of fetal restraint, see text relating to skin.

deformations and disruptions are brought about through the action of extrinsic processes, they are, by definition, not inherited. However, predisposition or sensitivity to certain extrinsic forces may be heritable.

The term "sequence" is used when a single anomaly of the fetus or its environment leads to a cascading series of defects. Thus, it implies an understanding of the pathogenesis leading to specific patterns of multiple anomalies. The fetal akinesia deformation sequence is a good example of such a cascade of developmental events, in which the lack of fetal movement acts as a common pathogenesis for a predictable sequence of structural defects, even though the etiology for the fetal akinesia can vary considerably (Moessinger, 1983). The fetal akinesia deformation sequence is schematically represented in Figure 1.

EFFECTS OF FETAL AKINESIA

The reduction or absence of fetal movement during a portion of gestation can result from any of a number of different etiologies (Figure 1). Regardless of how akinesia is produced, however, it acts as a common pathway in the development of different phenotypic outcomes. The diversity of effects produced by fetal akinesia is outlined in the following sections.

Congenital Contractures

Arthrogryposis (arthro: joint; grypos: curved), now usually called congenital contracture, is the permanent formation of a joint in a fixed position. There is a growing body of experimental evidence, beginning with the pioneering work of Drachman and Coulombre (1962), that demonstrates congenital contractures can result from immobilization of the joints during development (Swinyard & Bleck, 1985). Depending on the specific etiology of the akinesia and its timing during gestation, varying degrees of contracture can result. Different times of onset of akinesia also produce effects in different joints. In cases of spina bifida, for instance, usually only the lower extremities are affected. In cases of Werdnig-Hoffmann disease (infantile spinal muscular atrophy) of prenatal onset (with a generalized reduction in the number of anterior horn cells) most joints can be affected. The immobilization need not be permanent, however, for contractures to develop. Temporary paralysis induced experimentally has been demonstrated to produce contractures in chicken embryos (see Hofer; Provine, this volume). The effect of short-term paralysis in humans also has been suggested by a case involving a mother who had received tubocurarine for treatment of tetanus early in pregnancy (Jago, 1970). Tubocurarine is known to cross the placenta to the fetus, and in this case the baby was born with multiple congenital contractures. Thus the timing, duration and etiology of motor immobilization will affect the severity and the distribution of the contractures noted at birth.

One, many or all combinations of flexor and extensor contractures can occur, depending on the etiology of akinesia. Presumably, the exact nature of the contractures are affected by the position of the joints at the time of immobilization. Generally speaking, the long-term outcome will similarly depend on the etiology. If extrinsic fetal restraint is involved, most patients will recover near normal function after birth, given appropriate and early physical therapy. In contrast, if the cause for fetal immobilization persists postnatally, as occurs in the majority of cases involving myoneural dysfunction, the prognosis for full recovery to a normal range of motion is poor. Early recognition of the etiology underlying motor immobilization is essential in assessing recovery.

In many cases of congenital contractures with a myoneural etiology, the bones appear slender and thin. This probably reflects the absence or decrease in fetal movement that produces reduced mechanical force exerted on the growing bone. Muscle mass also can be markedly decreased in cases with denervation atrophy. In addition to the obvious effects of congenital contractions on motion, it should be emphasized that the normal ballistics of vaginal delivery can be jeopardized with such "nonpliant" fetuses, which can lead to some degree of intrapartum asphyxial injury. It is therefore important in newborn infants with congenital contractures and CNS dysfunction to distinguish the possible contribution of birth asphyxia to the CNS dysfunction from any other etiology.

Lung Hypoplasia

Hypoplasia denotes defective or incomplete development. Lung hypoplasia is a general term used to characterize lungs that are disproportionately small relative to body size and contain fewer cells or a reduced complement of DNA. Since the ability to breathe spontaneously at birth is critical for survival, newborn infants with severe lung hypoplasia tend to die early in the neonatal period. This condition is not rare and is currently recognized in one of seven perinatal autopsies. Although the precise pathogenesis responsible for the occurrence of lung hypoplasia remains unclear, a good deal of evidence points to the observation that fetal lung growth is mostly dependent on a single mechanical factor: stretch or distention of lung tissue. However, a major argument among fetal physiologists centers on how distention is exerted under normal circumstances.

Unless lung volume is maintained within normal limits, lung growth is disturbed. Lung volume in the fetus appears to be maintained by forces acting from within the organ itself (e.g., secretion or retention of fetal lung fluid), or by forces, both phasic and tonic, that expand the lung from the outside (fetal breathing and chest wall recoil). Several experiments with animal models have demonstrated the importance of these forces for lung growth. In humans, in cases of myoneural dysfunction where the absence of fetal .breathing movements has been documented by repeated ultrasound examination, the lungs were found to be hypoplastic. Fetal restraint, particularly when associated with (or resulting from) lack of amniotic fluid, frequently is associated with lung hypoplasia. Since fetal breathing activity is not markedly altered under these latter conditions (Moessinger et. al., 1987), suboptimal lung growth probably results from alterations in lung volume acting from within the lung itself (i.e., reduced fluid volume within the fetal lung). However, the precise mechanism by which oligohydramnios interferes with normal lung growth is poorly understood.

As is seen for the development of congenital contractures, timing of onset in gestation and duration of the insult play a role in the severity of the lesion, with early onset and prolonged duration associated with more severe outcome (Moessinger et. al., 1986). Sublethal forms of lung hypoplasia exist, and can contribute to perinatal asphyxia. Lung hypoplasia also may lead to postnatal hypoxia with some degree of CNS dysfunction, which will need to be distinguished from other, possibly inherited, disease entities.

Short Umbilical Cord

The length of the umbilical cord in newborn infants varies considerably. The broad distribution of measurements obtained is quite different from that recorded for any other fetal organ. Until recently, no significant correlation between cord length and other fetal or maternal characteristics had been documented. Recently, however, Smith and coworkers (Miller, Higginbottom & Smith, 1981) have provided evidence suggesting that umbilical cord length in humans is a reflection of fetal activity. Similarly, experiments with rat fetuses have demonstrated that longitudinal growth of the umbilical cord is determined, in part, by tensile forces produced by fetal activity, given adequate intrauterine space for movement (Moessinger, Blanc, Marone & Polsen, 1982). Pharmacological depression of fetal activity in rats results in shorter umbilical cords. The common association of polyhydramnios (which increases the intrauterine space available for fetal movement) and short umbilical cord in fetuses with myoneural dysfunction strongly supports the proposition that cord length is an indirect measure of fetal activity. Recognition that a short umbilical cord can be the consequence of early CNS dysfunction in the fetus will be of clinical importance, and perhaps medico-legal relevance as well. A short umbilical cord also can lead to asphyxial complications during a vaginal delivery. As with other anomalies discussed above, the search for a precise etiology of short umbilical cord is crucial for adequate long-term prognosis.

Facial Anomalies

Of the many anomalies in facial morphology encountered in patients with either myoneural dysfunction or fetal restraint, several are observed only in a small subset of patients. This restricted occurrence is probably dependent on the exact cause of fetal akinesia. The common features encountered in the fetal akinesia deformation sequence include micrognathia (frequently associated with a small mouth), low set ears, small alae nasae and, frequently, some degree of hypertelorism (wide distance between the eyes). Fetal restraint produced by external compression obviously can mold the face in many ways, depending on the position of the fetus within the uterus and the direction of the compressive forces. Likewise, the growth of the brain in size has a direct effect on the growth of the calvarium, which in turn affects the appearance of facial features. Patients with either marked microcephaly or massive hydrocephaly have distinct but characteristic facial features. In addition to the mechanical impact of brain development and skull growth on facial form, indirect effects of neuromuscular function on facial development have been recognized (Smith, 1981). It is of considerable interest to note that the facial features associated with the fetal akinesia deformation sequence are also the hallmark of the Moebius malformation sequence (congenital facial diplegia or paralysis). It thus appears that these facial features develop secondary to a deficit in facial muscle contractions during fetal development.

Growth Deficiency

When born close to term, most infants subjected to depressed activity in utero weigh less than expected for their gestational age. A notable exception to this rule are infants with oligohydramnios that resulted from early membrane rupture. As mentioned above, bones appear thinner in many cases of arthrogryposis with a myoneural etiology. In cases with denervation atrophy, muscle mass is markedly decreased. Although these examples suggest that fetal motor activity is essential for normal weight gain, little data are available to firmly establish this point. To my knowledge, studies of the relative mass of different compartments of the body are lacking.

Microgastria

There is a remarkable paucity of information on gut development in cases of fetal akinesia. In an animal model of akinesia induced by fetal curarization (Moessinger, 1983), small stomachs were noted. These experiments with fetal rats further demonstrated that the polyhydramnios associated with fetal akinesia was the result of impaired swallowing of amniotic fluid by the fetus. Additional experiments involving induction of oligohydramnios in fetal rats resulted in shortened gut length. Blanc, Apperson and McNally (1962) noted microgastria in half of their patients with the oligohydramnios deformation sequence. In unrelated cases with intestinal atresia, while the proximal segment of the intestine tends to be dilated, the distal segment is usually small in caliber. This effect possibly expresses the influence of intraluminal distending forces. But very few studies have focused on this aspect of fetal development.

Skin

According to Smith (1981), the skin does not appear to have any basic impetus for growth, but rather grows in response to the application of mechanical force. Intrinsic mechanical force is usually exerted by the growth or movement of underlying tissues. As a consequence of reduced cutaneous growth, the skin usually appears tight and thin in most cases with myoneural dysfunction. This observation is particularly evident around the fixed joints, where occasional webs of tight skin on the flexor surface can be demonstrated by attempting to extend the joint. In contrast, in most cases with extrinsic fetal constraint, the skin often appears thick and loose, and exhibits abundant folds. The simplest explanation for the apparent discrepancy between the effects of intrinsic and extrinsic immobilization is that skin growth responds to external pressure or stretch in a similar fashion to its response to internal expansile stretch. For example, when a fetus with an intact neuromuscular system is restrained by lack of amniotic fluid, its attempts to move are likely to stretch the skin resting in direct contact with the wall of the uterine cavity; the result is excess skin with abundant folds. In contrast, a fetus with myoneural dysfunction and therefore reduced development of underlying muscle tissue, experiences less internal force to stretch the skin, with consequent thinning and tightening of the skin.

PROBLEMS IN INTERPRETING PATHOGENESIS

While it is usually held that the pathogenesis for the oligohydramnios deformation sequence is "fetal compression", I tend to disagree with this view and would suggest that fetal restraint plays a key role. The best example to illustrate this interpretation is the twin-to-twin transfusion-syndrome. When identical twins share one placenta (monochorionic), but have two distinct amniotic sacs, vascular anastomoses between the fetuses are common. When anastomosis is arterio-venous in type, as a result of the pressure gradient between artery and vein, one fetus (donor) will tend to transfuse blood to the other (recipient). The donor may develop prerenal oliguria with resultant oligohydramnios while the recipient often develops polyhydramnios. If this situation persists over weeks, the fetus with oligohydramnios will display all the features of the oligohydramnios deformation sequence while the other fetus will either be normal with some degree of polycythemia or display signs of heart failure (induced by fluid overload) with hydrops.

In the situation of twin-to-twin transfusion syndrome, both fetuses develop within the same uterus and are separated only by a thin diamniotic membrane. Therefore, both fetuses are subjected to similar amounts of intrauterine pressure or compression. It appears likely that the reduction of amniotic fluid in the amniotic sac of the donor fetus is effective in restricting its range of motion. Thus, restriction of movement, and not fetal compression, appears responsible for the deformation sequence.

CONCLUDING REMARKS

In this essay I have briefly presented some of the evidence supporting the general concept that fetal activity is an important determinant of normal morphological development. Until recently, it was technically difficult, if not impossible, to gather information on normal fetal activity. With the current development of techniques for ultrasonic imaging of human fetuses in utero (Prechtl, 1985; also see Birnholz, this volume), and the direct study of nonhuman fetuses (see Smotherman & Robinson, this volume), we stand to learn a great deal about embryonic and fetal activity and how it evolves with advancing gestational age. Only with this understanding will we be in a position to properly define the morphological correlates of normal or abnormal fetal activity.

References

Blanc, W. A., Apperson, J. W., & Mcnally, J. (1962). Pathology of the newborn and of the placenta in oligohydramnios. *Bulletin of Sloane Hospital, 8,* 51−64.

Drachman, B. B., & Coulombre, A. J. (1962). Experimental clubfoot and arthrogryposis multiplex congenita. *Lancet, 2,* 523−526.

Dunn, P. M. (1976). Congenital postural deformities. *British Medical Bulletin, 32,* 71−76.

Jago, R. H. (1970). Arthrogryposis following treatment of maternal tetanus with muscle relaxants. *Archives of Diseases of Children, 45,* 277−279.

Lamarck, J. B. (1809). *Philosophie zoologique.* Paris: Dentu.

Miller, M. E., Higginbottom, M., & Smith, D. W. (1981). Short umbilical cord: its origin and relevance. *Pediatrics, 67,* 618−621.

Moessinger, A. C. (1983). Fetal akinesia deformation sequence: an animal model. *Pediatrics, 72,* 857−863.

Moessinger, A. C., Blanc, W. A., Marone, P. A., & Polsen, D. C. (1982). Umbilical cord length as an index of fetal activity: experimental study and clinical implications. *Pediatric Research, 16,* 109−112.

Moessinger, A. C., Collins, M. H., Blanc, W. A., Rey, H. R., & James, L. S. (1986). Oligohydramnios-induced lung hypoplasia: the influence of timing and duration in gestation. *Pediatric Research, 20,* 951−954.

Moessinger, A. C., Fox, H. E., Higgins, A., Rey, H. R. & Al Haideri, M. (1987) Fetal breathing movements are not a reliable predictor of continued lung development in pregnancies complicated by oligohydramnios *Lancet, 2,* 1297−1300.

Prechtl, H. F. R., (Ed.). (1985). (Special issue on ultrasound studies of human fetal behaviour.) *Early Human Development, 12,* 91−209.

Smith, D. W. (1981). Mechanics in morphogenesis: principles and response of particular tissues. In *Recognizable patterns of human deformation, Vol. 21, Major problems in clinical pediatrics,* (pp. 110−144). New York: W. B. Saunders.

Spranger, J., Benirschke, K., Hall, J. G., Lenz, W., Lowry, R. B., Opitz, J. M., Pinsky, L., Schwarzacher, H. G., & Smith, D. W. (1982). Errors of morphogenesis: concepts and terms. Recommendations of an international working group. *Journal of Pediatrics, 100,* 160−165.

Swinyard, C. A., & Bleck, E. (1985). The etiology of arthrogryposis (multiple congenital contracture). *Clinical Orthopaedics, 194,* 15−29.

Thompson, D. W. (1942). *On growth and form.* Cambridge: Cambridge University Press.

Auditory Experience in the Fetus

William P. Fifer and Christine Moon
Department of Developmental Psychobiology
New York State Psychiatric Institute
Columbia University
New York, New York

In order to explore and understand the forces that shape early cognitive, social and emotional processes, increasing numbers of researchers are eavesdropping on the fetus. Special attention to the form and function of *in utero* experience, particularly with the maternal voice, has raised important research questions regarding the evolving interaction between the fetus and the maternal environment. Growing interest within several disciplines concerning the psychobiological significance of prenatal auditory experience and the continued development of more sophisticated techniques now allow these issues to be systematically investigated.

SOUND IN THE FETAL ENVIRONMENT AND EARLY AUDITORY RESPONSIVENESS

Several investigators have succeeded in making *in utero* recordings by inserting a small hydrophone or microphone into the amniotic cavity near the fetus' head. This has been done with humans after rupture of the amniotic membranes during labor (Bench, 1973; Henschall, 1972; Murooka, Koie & Suda, 1976; Querleu & Renard, 1981; Versyp, 1985) and with sheep over a period of weeks prior to birth (Vince, Billing, Baldwin, Toner & Weller, 1985). There is agreement among researchers that the fetal acoustic environment is a rich one. The human maternal pulse is audible as well as borborygmi from digestion. In addition, very low frequency noise has been reported which may be related to the maternal vascular system, but is in the frequency range below human hearing. Mother's voice is a prominent sound in the amniotic environment, is not substantially masked by other sounds, and represents a stronger signal than external voices. All voice signals are altered by transmission through maternal tissue and amniotic fluid, resulting in a progressive attenuation of frequencies above 1000 Hz.

However, much remains to be described about the acoustic nature of mother's voice in the intrauterine cavity. Recent recordings estimate background vascular noise to be about 30dB at 300Hz, which is the region of the first formant frequency for most adult women's voices. At 300Hz the maternal voice signal has been reported to be between 40 to 50 dB (Versyp, 1985). Investigators are generally in agreement that sounds are progressively attenuated at higher frequencies beginning at about 500Hz. There is still a question, however, as to the degree of attenuation. In the most recent and technically sophisticated study of sound recorded *in utero*, frequencies were detected in higher ranges than had been previously reported (Versyp, 1985). Furthermore, animal and human studies are somewhat at variance. Acoustic recordings in humans have been limited to the period after rupture of membranes during labor, which means that some fluid has drained out of the amniotic cavity, and that the microphone is inserted into a constricted area next to the fetal head. Human studies typically report more powerful acoustic stimuli with more distortion of outside voices than animal studies in which it is possible to make recordings over a longer period of time prior to labor. Versyp (1985) found that adult recognition of intrauterine recordings of nonsense syllables was less than 50% overall. But Vince and coworkers (1985) reported "perfectly audible" and "usually distinct" words of outside voices in their intrauterine sheep recordings. Recording conditions and task, as well as anatomical differences between humans and sheep, probably account for the disparity. The question remains unanswered as to the intactness of the speech signal *in utero*.

Given that the acoustic signal *in utero* can eventually be accurately described, there remains the difficult problem of measuring fetal perception of pitch and loudness. For example, fluid is the medium of transmission in both the outer and middle ear of the fetus, and it is not known how this affects the acoustic signal prior to reaching the basilar membrane, which itself is undergoing change throughout the third trimester (Rubel, 1985). Much of what can be said about human prenatal audition must await advances in the psychophysics of the fetus. However, fetal responsiveness to several types of extramaternal acoustic signals has been documented, indicating at the very least an ability to detect sounds.

Thorough reviews of the development of the fetal auditory system can be found in Pujol and Hilding (1973), Rubel (1985), and Lecanuet, Granier-Deferre & Busnel (submitted). There is a literature dating back to Peiper (1925) and Forbes and Forbes (1927) demonstrating fetal responsiveness to auditory stimuli. Fetal heart rate changes have been observed to externally presented pure tones as early as 24 weeks gestational age (Bernard and Sontag, 1947; Sontag & Wallace, 1936) and eye blinks following vibroacoustic stimulation were recorded in a 25 week old fetus (Birnholz & Benaceraf, 1983; see also Birnholz, this volume). More recently, standardized acoustic vibratory stimuli have been used to assess fetal reactivity and to characterize state changes in the fetus (Gagnon, Hunse, Carmichael, Fellows & Patrick, 1987). Recent advances in ultrasound imaging have allowed observations of global body and limb movement to external sounds (Gelman, Wood, Spellacy and Abrams, 1982; Leader, Baillie, Martin and Vermuelen, 1982). Jensen (1984) has demonstrated that changes in fetal cardiac response occur as early as 32 weeks and then begin to increase as a function of gestational age. Additional indirect evidence for early fetal auditory capabilities come from studies suggesting that premature infants will show evoked cortical and cardiac responding to some types of auditory stimulation between 24 and 29 weeks gestational age and will respond behaviorally to a wide variety of sounds by 34 weeks of age (Als, Lester, and Brazelton, 1979; Parmalee, 1981; Starr, Amlie, Martin and Sanders, 1977). Thus, the human fetus appears to have an intact, well-developed auditory system by the final trimester of gestation and has had considerable opportunity to sample from a rich acoustic environment.

FUNCTION OF PRENATAL EXPERIENCE

Neural Development

The experience with external sounds may serve a role of enrichment or fine tuning of the fetal auditory system, (Gottlieb, 1985; Lecanuet et al., submitted). Moreover, the developing system, with low frequency sensitivity emerging first, may be making optimal use of the available stimuli. Rubel (1985) notes that the transmission of sounds favoring low frequencies, while attenuating high frequencies, parallels auditory neuronal development. The early sculpting of neuronal circuitry underlying the development of hemispheric specialization may be tied to developmental changes in sound transmission resulting from changes in the shape and density of the maternal abdominal wall, relative amount of amniotic fluid, and fetal head position throughout pregnancy (Turkewitz, in press). It is important to consider that the role these experiences play in the shaping of neural function may not be limited to the auditory system (Greenough, Black and Wallace, 1987). For example, the coupling of auditory stimulation with the sensations resulting from movement of the mother's diaphragm while talking, may not only serve to make maternal speech more salient, but can provide an important source of contingent and multimodal experience for the fetus. Moreover, experience with auditory events may serve as one of the primary forces participating in the organization of several integrated neural patterns underlying newborn sensory and perceptual preferences. Presumably, some neural predispositions exist for the late-term fetus which were in fact shaped by prenatal auditory experience during even earlier periods of fetal development.

Speech Perception and Voice Recognition

One of the most direct influences of prenatal auditory experience may be on newborn speech perception and voice recognition. The voice signal, especially that of mother, is likely to have increased salience for the fetus relative to other auditory events. Mother's speech signal in the womb differs from other sounds in its intensity, variability, and multimodal character. Mother's voice has been reported to be the most intense acoustic signal measured in the amniotic environment, dominating vascular, digestive, and extramaternal sounds (Versyp, 1985). Vascular sounds are relatively invariant in rhythm, although they may vary in loudness depending upon how close the fetal ear is to the uterine vessels. Researchers have obtained different maternal vascular system acoustic intensity readings depending upon the location of the intrauterine microphone (Vince et al., 1985). It is not known how frequently the fetus experiences maternal digestive sounds, or borborygmi. They do not, however, mask the maternal voice. Moreover, while borborygmi are variable in pitch and rhythm and may provide some fetal stimulation from coincident tissue movement, the diaphragm muscle movement accompanying mother's voice is likely to result in a greater amount of kinesthetic and tactile stimulation than that associated with other sounds. The conjugate, multimodal, and perhaps more arousing nature of this stimulation may promote greater fetal responsivity to the maternal voice than to any other prenatal sound.

The component of maternal speech with which the developing fetus probably has the most experience is prosody: the intonation, stress, and rhythm of language. Prosody is carried by the frequencies which are reportedly the least attenuated in the prenatal environment. Morever, the stress and rhythm of prosody would presumably be accompanied by maternal diaphragm movements, giving conjugate stimulation. There is strong evidence that the prosodic characteristics of speech are attended to by young infants (Fernald, 1985; Mehler, Bertoncini, Barriere & Jassik-Gerschenfeld, 1987), possibly as a result of prenatal experience. Prosody is the characteristic of the speech signal most likely to remain constant from fetal to newborn life. It may be the basis of two-day-olds' ability to recognize mother's voice (DeCasper & Fifer, 1980; Fifer & Moon, submitted). That it is possible to recognize familiar voices on the basis of prosodic information alone has been demonstrated in adults (Abberton & Fourcin, 1978).

A fetal predisposition to attend to the prosodic elements of speech could also serve the function of providing the newborn with the basis for acquisition of information about caretaker emotional state. Pitch, stress, rhythm, and intonation are carriers of cues to emotional state. Empathy, an integral component of emotion, may be present at birth, and attention to prosody may be an important cue for infants in the earliest stages of emotional development (Campos, Barrett, Lamb, Goldsmith & Stenberg, 1983).

Evidence for prenatal exposure to the non-prosodic elements of the speech signal is not as clear as for the prosodic elements. It is not known how much information about speech segments is transmitted into the intrauterine environment. Such information is carried by frequencies which have been reported to be greatly attenuated in transmission through maternal tissue and amniotic fluid. In one experiment, fetuses reportedly evinced discrimination of a change in order of vowel presentation (Lecanuet, Busnel, DeCasper, Granier-Deferre, & Maugeais, 1986). Vowel identification requires more information than is available in those frequencies which presumably remain unattenuated *in utero*. Two-day-old infants discriminate order of consonants (Moon, 1985) and four to five-day-olds discriminate between very brief syllables differing only in onset properties (Bertoncini, Bijeljac-Babic, Blumstein, & Mehler, 1987). Whether these very early capacities benefit from prenatal experience is not known. It does appear, however, that the salience of segmental portions of the speech signal increases as infants approach the end of the first year. Not until around the age of 10 months do infants show a differential sensitivity to segments unique to their language environment (Werker, Gilbert, Humphrey & Tees, 1981). Relative lack of prenatal exposure to segmental as compared to prosodic properties of speech may predispose newborns to selectively attend to prosody, even though they have the capacity to differentiate segmental units.

It is now within the scope of current research methods to investigate more directly the effect on the fetus of prenatal exposure to the speech signal. As Lecanuet and others (Lecanuet, Granier-Deferre, Cohen, Le Houezec, & Busnel, 1986) have shown, it is possible to obtain differential responding in fetuses to sounds of speech. With expected advances in fetal recording it should be possible to more fully characterize the developing salience and discrimination of both prosodic and segmental aspects of speech.

Cognitive Development

The demonstration at birth that infants are capable of learning a discrimination task which enables access to recordings of different voices indicates the presence of a mechanism available during the perinatal period for acquiring associations between environmental events. This suggests that both the fetus and the newborn are even more competent learners than is usually believed. In fact, DeCasper and Spence (1986), Panneton (1985), and Satt (1985) have reported data indicating that newborns may be able to demonstrate a postnatal preference for a specific melody or passage experienced prenatally.

These investigations into the development of auditory preferences may lead to a better understanding of the development of early learning capabilities. For example, how do infants learn to organize their behavior around the distinctive features of the caretaker? The fetus has been introduced to a portion of these distinctive auditory features during the last weeks of gestation. What is the nature of the stimuli with which the fetus becomes familiar? What exactly does the fetus remember? Finally, what is the context in which these stimuli are experienced? The latter, in fact, may be the critical dimension on which to focus investigations into prenatal auditory learning, because it is the context in which an event occurs that in large measure determines the representation of that event in memory (Balsam, 1985). Moreover, the multimodal and presumably highly arousing stimulation received by the fetus during maternal speech may also have an impact on early learning mechanisms by playing a role in facilitating and maintaining periods of alert activity during which the fetus explores and learns about the context of the *in utero* environment. A more thorough characterization of the fetal auditory experience should help in our explorations of several other learning issues as well, including the origins of the orienting response, and the importance of state and level of arousal on early learning and memory.

Social/Emotional Development

The investigation of the origins of the attachment process has recently focused on the perinatal period. As pointed out by Hofer (this volume) an effective network of maternal regulators is well established at birth and the complex interactions between mother and infant have begun. Research in early attachment indicates that newborns differentially respond to, interact with, and actively seek contact with a wide range of proximal "maternal" stimuli, (e.g., odor, touch, visual stimulation). However, the infant's proximity-seeking behaviors serve to establish not only early proximal interactions, but later in development, more distal interactions such as maintaining eye contact, smiling or following. Moreover, a differential sensitivity in the newborn to such distal cues (i.e., listening to the caretaker's voice from a distance) may more directly subserve later attachment behaviors, which primarily consist of the toddler's responses to maternal presence or absence in the auditory or visual field. Thus, the development of the reciprocal interactions essential in the earliest stages of the attachment process may be facilitated by early discrimination and preference for mother's voice.

Fetal experience with mother's voice, in addition to providing a substrate for early social processes, may also support early emotional development. Current theories of emotion describe "primordial" responses which have hedonic value, are relatively stimulus-bound, and are biologically adaptive (Barrett & Campos, 1987). For example, the "savoring" sucking patterns exhibited by newborns upon experiencing sweet taste (Lipsitt, 1979), and distress behavior evoked by abrupt onset of visual or auditory stimuli have been offered as examples of primordial or "hardwired" emotions. One measure of positive hedonic value in young infants is the willingness to approach a stimulus. Approach responses have been recorded to familiar olfactory stimuli such as maternal breast milk (MacFarlane, 1975) and axillary odor (Cernoch & Porter, 1985). Selective neonatal responses to familiar prenatal sounds include changing sucking patterns to activate sounds experienced *in utero* (DeCasper & Sigafoos, 1983; Moon & Fifer, 1986) and calming during a recording of intrauterine heartbeat sounds (Murooka, et al., 1976; Rosner & Doherty, 1971). These responses to olfactory and auditory stimuli appear to qualify as examples of primordial emotion in that they reflect hedonic value and could be interpreted as promoting the neonate's survival through maintenance of contact with the source of sustenance.

In addition, approach responses have been documented to stimuli that are not as universal and consistent as sweet tastes or abrupt onsets or as clearly sustenance-related as mother's milk or womb sounds. Various stimuli appear to acquire positive value through repeated exposure. Examples are cherry or white ginger odor placed in the bassinets of neonates (Balogh & Porter, 1986), a story read prenatally (DeCasper & Spence, 1986), a melody sung prenatally (Panneton, 1985), and the sound of the newborn's own mother's voice either reading (DeCasper & Fifer, 1980) or in adult conversation (Fifer & Moon, submitted). Newborns may exhibit a pattern of preference for familiarity that has been documented elsewhere. In children and adults, mere exposure to auditory stimuli has been described as sufficient to generate a preference for those sounds even though the preferred stimuli may not be recognized as familiar. The effect has been proposed as evidence that emotional and cognitive capacities are separable (Zajonc, 1980; 1984).

If sounds which have acquired positive hedonic value through repeated exposure are admitted into the category of primordial emotional stimuli, then emotional experiences are likely to begin prior to birth. The early preference for the sound of mother's voice may be evidence for this. Further support of the notion lies in the observation that emotional responses originate in phylogenetically and ontogenetically older parts of the brain (Zajonc, 1984), structures which are relatively more developed in the third trimester fetus than sites for cognitive processing. The selective response to mother's voice may be an emotional preference which is limited to similar stimuli. There is some evidence for this. The sound of an unfamiliar female voice is reinforcing to newborns (Fifer & Moon, submitted) but an unfamiliar male voice is not (DeCasper & Prescott, 1984) or only weakly reinforcing (Moon & Fifer, 1988). Male voices, which are lower in frequency, may be masked by low frequency intra-uterine sounds and not as available to the fetus as non-maternal female voices (DeCasper & Prescott, 1984). Alternatively, the stronger approach response to unfamiliar female voices could result from a generalization of a preference for mother's voice. For either explanation, differential responsiveness, indicated by activation of the voice through changes in infant sucking patterns, implies differential positive hedonic value, prob-ably accrued prenatally, for the newborn.

METHODOLOGICAL ISSUES

The method for measurement of newborn auditory discrimination, based on differential contingent sucking patterns, has now been used to demon-strate a preference for mother's voice over silence, for female voice over silence, and for mother's voice over other female voices (DeCasper & Fifer, 1980; Fifer & Moon, submitted). Variations of the same technique have been used to show that a version of mother's voice altered to approximate uterine characteristics is preferred to a normal recording of her voice (Moon & Fifer, submitted; Spence & DeCasper, 1987). Such assessments of differential responsiveness in the newborn to prenatal and postnatal versions of sounds should continue to be useful for investigating capacities and predispositions acquired in utero.

Several researchers are using directional changes in heart rate to inves-tigate fetal and newborn responsiveness to sounds. There is a growing body of research with infants examining the relationship between individual differences in heart rate variability and responsiveness to a wide range of environmental stimuli (Clifton, 1974; Porges, Arnold, & Forbes, 1973). Heart rate variability can be decomposed into several rhythmic periodicities. The most extensively investigated component of heart rate variability, respiratory sinus arrhythmia (RSA), is mediated by cyclical changes in vagal nerve activity and thus is used to quantify parasympathetic influences on the heart (see Porges, McCabe & Yongue, 1982, for a review of this literature). Porges and others have used this variable as an index of central nervous system integrity and as a predictor variable for later assessment of attention and cognitive maturation (Fox & Porges, 1985; Richards, 1985). These estimates of autonomic function appear to be very sensitive to individual differences in responsiveness to environmental stimuli. Several researchers contend that this reactivity does not simply reflect a quantification of the orienting response, but a more complicated process involving sampling from the environment and evaluation for stimulus significance (Coles, 1984; Porges et al., 1973). Recently, RSA has been used as a dependent measure of the acute response to auditory stimulation in newborns (Fifer, Monti, Myers & Yongue, 1986). This ability to more fully characterize differential autonomic responses to auditory stimulation will enable questions to be asked regarding relative familiarity with different speech signals (Fifer et al., 1986). Using similar measures to characterize autonomic responding in the fetus, it may be possible to assess differential responding to familiar and unfamiliar prenatal stimuli.

   Although using heart rate variability as a dependent measure of re-sponsiveness is a relatively new approach, it can provide a more rich quantification of both newborn and fetal autonomic activity than do more traditional analyses of directional heart rate change. However, as with the behavioral discrimination procedures, these autonomic measures appear to be significantly modulated by state. There is a large literature on exploration of heart rate responsiveness during various sleep states and attention to state issues has enhanced reliability and validity of all newborn data (Berg & Berg, 1982; Campos & Brackbill, 1973; Jusczyk, 1985). The effect of sleep/wake states must be a primary consideration in any future investigation of the autonomic response of the perinate to speech sounds. Furthermore, there is a need for more data on the effect of state on the kind of "higher cognitive activity" which may be involved in the preferential response to speech signals or in voice recognition.

   Additionally, since the fetus spends much of the time in active-sleep (paradoxical, REM), it may be important to characterize its response to the presentation of salient stimuli in this state. That is, what effect does speech have on the sleeping fetus? Has it some impact on early organization of states or elicitation of evolving components of sleep states? Does the fetus habituate or change state during various periods of maternal speech stimulation? Are there individual differences in the occurrence and maintenance of different fetal states during speech, as we observe with newborns? Does a fetus respond differentially to the speech frequencies associated with levels of stress in adults? In newborns, lower frequency sounds may be better inhibitors of infant distress, and high frequencies (above 400 Hz) tend to occasion distress (Eisenberg, 1976). Such perinatal sensitivities could have an impact on the early emergence of the emotional states referred to by Hofer (this volume) that are tied to the physiological functions essential for survival. Recognizing that the development of most of the processes labeled cognitive, social and emotional may in large measure depend on prenatal tuning of physiological response systems, the answers to these questions may initially depend on our ability to characterize early markers of emotional and cognitive reactivity (e.g., cardiovascular responsiveness). Finally, though the fetal environment and psychobiological systems are undergoing rapid change, measurement of both autonomic and behavioral responses, in different states and at different ages, should combine to create more sensitive measures for detection of the developmental course and consequences of fetal auditory experience.

SUMMARY

Over the past decade evidence has accumulated that experience with sounds begins prior to birth. Experience with sound in the womb is likely to contribute in important ways both to fetal and newborn development. The acoustic environment of the fetus is rich with sounds of the maternal vascular system, borborygmi, externally transmitted noises and voices, and most prominently, mother's voice. Little is known about how the developing fetus perceives the available sound, although fetal responsiveness to a variety of external sounds has been documented. This early experience has likely ramifications for neural development, speech perception and voice recognition, as well as cognitive, emotional and social growth. Although problems with state lability and limited access to subjects requires a relatively large time investment, we believe the resulting data will (a) significantly contribute to the body of knowledge on fetal sensory, perceptual and behavioral development, (b) increase our understanding of the effects of fetal experience, maturation and state on responsiveness to external stimulation, (c) further specify the nature of the "psychobiological" environment of the fetus, (d) offer data which may guide effective assessments of fetal well-being, and (e) provide a set of techniques and a framework for studying the development of other fetal capabilities.

Acknowledgements

We would like to thank Peter Balsam for his thoughtful comments on a previous version of this manuscript. We also are grateful to Lisa Monti and Catherine Raeff for their aid in preparing and editing the manuscript. Preparation of this manuscript and much of the research was supported by the Research Foundation for Mental Hygiene, the New York State Psychiatric Institute and a grant from the National Institute of Child Health and Human Development (HD20102).

References

Abberton, E. & Fourcin, A. J. (1978) Intonation and speaker identification. *Language and Speech, 21*, 305–318.

Als, H., Lester, M. B., & Brazelton, T. B. (1979) Dynamics of the behavioral organization of the premature infant: A theoretical perspective. In T. Field, S. Goldberg, A. Sostek, & H. Shuman (Eds.), *The High Risk Newborn*. New York: Spectrum.

Balogh, R. D. & Porter, R. H. (1986) Olfactory preferences resulting from mere exposure in human neonates. *Infant Behavior and Development, 9*, 395–401.

Balsam, P. D. (1985) The functions of context in learning and performance. In P. D. Balsam & A. Tomie, (Eds.) *Context and Learning*. Hillsdale: Lawrence Erlbaum Associates.

Barrett, K. C. & Campos, J. J. (1987) Perspectives on emotional development II: A functionalist approach to emotions. In J. D. Osofsky (Ed.), *Handbook of Infant Development*. New York: Wiley.

Bench, J. (1973) Fetal audiometry in relation to the developing fetal nervous system. In W. Taylor (Ed.) *Disorders of Auditory Function*. London and New York: Academic Press.

Berg, W. K. & Berg, K. M. (1980) Psychophysiological development in infancy: state, sensory function, and attention. In J. Osofsky (Ed.), *Handbook of Infant Development*. New York: Wiley.

Bernard, J., & Sontag, L. W. (1947) Fetal reactivity to tonal stimulation: A preliminary report. *Journal of Genetic Psychology, 70*, 205–210.

Bertoncini, J., Bijeljac-Babic, R., Blumstein, S., & Mehler, J. (1987) Discrimination in neonates of very short CVs. *Journal of the Acoustic Society of America, 82*, 31–37.

Birnholz, J. C. & Benaceraff, B. B. (1983) The development of fetal hearing. *Science, 222*, 516-518.

Campos, J. J., Barrett, K. C., Lamb, M. E., Goldsmith, H. H., & Stenberg, C. (1983). Socioemotional development. In P. H. Mussen (Ed.), *Handbook of Child Psychology*. New York: Wiley.

Campos, J. J. & Brackbill, Y. (1973) Infant state: relationship to heart rate, behavioral response and response decrement. *Developmental Psychobiology, 6*, 9–19.

Cernoch, J. M., & Porter, R. H. (1985) Recognition of maternal axillary odors by infants. *Child Development*, *56*, 1593−1598.

Clifton, R. (1974) Heart rate conditioning in the newborn infant. *Journal of Experimental Child Psychology*, *18*, 9−21.

Coles, M. G. H. (1984) Heart rate and attention: The intake-rejection hypothesis and beyond. In M. G. H. Coles, J. R. Jennings and J. A. Stern (Eds.), *Psychological Perspectives*. New York: van Nostrand Reinhold

DeCasper, A. J., & Fifer, W. P. (1980) Of human boding: Newborns prefer their mothers' voices. *Science*, *208*, 1174−1176.

DeCasper, A. J. & Prescott, A. (1984). Human newborns perception of male voices: Preference, discrimination, and reinforcing value. *Developmental Psychobiology*, *17*, 481− 491.

DeCasper, A. J., & Sigafoos, A. D. (1983). The intrauterine heartbeat: A potent reinforcer for newborns. *Infant Behavior and Development*, *6*, 19−25.

DeCasper, A. J., & Spence, M. (1986). Newborns prefer a familiar story over an unfamiliar one. *Infant Behavior and Development*, *9*, 133−150.

Eisenberg, R. B. (1976) *Auditory competence in early life: The roots of communicative behavior*. Baltimore: University Park Press.

Fernald, A. (1985) Four-month old infants prefer to listen to motherese. *Infant Behavior and Development*, *8*, 181−195.

Fifer, W. P., Monti, L. M., Myers M. M., & Yongue, B. (1986) Autonomic response to mother's voice in the newborn. Paper presented at Annual Meeting of the International Society for Development Psychobiology, Annapolis, November.

Fifer, W. P., & Moon, C. (1988) Newborn discrimination learning: The value of voices. Manuscript submitted for publication.

Forbes, H. S., & Forbes, H. B. (1927) Fetal sense reaction: hearing. *Journal of Comparative Physiological Psychology*, *7*, 353−355.

Fox, N. L., & Porges, S. W. (1985) The relationship between developmental outcome and neonatal heart rate pattern. *Child Development*, *56*, 28−37.

Gagnon, R., Hunse, C., Carmichael, L., Fellows, F., & Patrick, J. (1987) External vibratory acoustic stimulation near term: Fetal heart rate and heart rate variability responses. *American Journal of Obstetrics and Gynecology*, *156*, 323−327.

Gelman, S. R., Wood, S., Spellacy, W. N., & Abrams, R. M. (1982) Fetal movements in response to sound stimulation. *American Journal Obstetrics Gynecology*, *143*, 484−485.

Gottlieb, G. (1985) On discovering significant acoustic dimensions of auditory stimulation for infants. In G. Gotlieb & N. A. Krasnegor (Eds.), *Measurement of Audition and Vision in the First Year of Postnatal Life: A Methodological Overview*. Norwood, N. J.: Ablex.

Greenough, W. T., Black, J. E., & Wallace, C. S. (1987) Experience and brain development. *Child Development*, *58*, 3, 539−559.

Henschall, W. R. (1972) Intrauterine sound levels. *Journal of Obstetrics and Gynecology*, *112*, 577−579.

Jensen, O. H. (1984) Fetal heart rate response to controlled sound stimuli during the third trimester of normal pregnancy, *Acta Obstetric Gynecol Scand.*, *63*, 193−197.

Jusczyk, P. W. (1985) The high-amplitude sucking technique as a methodological tool in speech perception research, In G. Gottlieb & N. A. Krasnegor (Eds.), *Measurement of Audition and Vision in the First Year of Postnatal Life: A Methodological Overview*. Norwood, NJ: Ablex.

Leader, L. R., Baillie, P., Martin, B., & Vermuelen, E. (1982) The assessment and significance of habituation to a repeated stimulus by the human fetus. *Early Human Development*, *7*, 211−219.

Lecanuet, J-P., Busnel, M-C., DeCasper, A. J., Granier-Deferre, C., & Maugeais, R. (1986) Familiar and unfamiliar speech elicit different cardiac responses in human fetuses. Paper presented at the meeting of the International Society for Developmental Psychobiology, Annapolis, November 6–9.

Lecanuet, J-P., Granier-Deferre, C., Collen, H., Houezec, R., & Busnel, M-C. (1986) Fetal response to acoustic stimulation depends on heartrate variability pattern, stimulus intensity and repetition. *Early Human Development, 13* 269–283.

Lecanuet, J-P., Granier-Deferre, C., & Busnel, M-C. (1988) L' Audition prenatale. Manuscript submitted for publication.

Lipsitt, L. P. (1979) The pleasures and annoyances of infants: Approach and avoidance behavior. In E. Thoman (Ed.), *Origins of infants' social responsiveness.* Hillsdale, NJ: Erlbaum.

MacFarlane, A. (1975) Olfaction in the development of social preferences in the human neonate. *Ciba Foundation Symposium, 33,* 103–117.

Mehler, J., Bertoncini, J., Barriere, M., & Jassik-Gershenfeld, D. (1987) Infant recognition of mother's voice. *Perception, 7,* 491–497.

Moon, C. (1985) Phonological universals and syllable discrimination in one-to three-day old infants. Columbia University doctoral dissertation. Ann Arbor: University Microfilms International.

Moon, C., & Fifer, W. P. (1986) Newborns prefer the sound of mother's voice as experienced in the womb. Paper presented at International Society for Developmental Psychobiology, Annual Meeting, Annapolis, November.

Moon, C. and Fifer, W. P. (1988) Newborn response to a male voice. Poster presented at biannual meeting of International Conference on Infant studies, Washington, D. C., May.

Murooka, H., Koie, I., & Suda, D. (1976) Analyse des sons intrauterines et de leurs effects tranquillisants sur le nouveau-ne. *Journal de de Gynecologie, Obstetrique, et Biologie de la Reproduction, 5,* 367–376.

Panneton, R. P. (1985) Prenatal experience with melodies: Effect on postnatal auditory preference in human newborns. Unpublished doctoral dissertation, University of North Carolina at Greensboro.

Parmelee, A. H. (1981) Auditory function and neurological maturation in premature infants. In S. Friedman & M. Sigman (Eds.) *Preterm Birth and Psychological Development.* New York: Academic Press.

Peiper, A. (1925) Sinnesempfindungen des Kindes vor seiner Geburt. *Msr. Kinderheik, 29,* 236.

Porges, S. W., Arnold W. R., & Forbes, E. J. (1973) Heart rate variability: an index of attentional responsivity in human newborns. *Developmental Psychology, 8,* 85–92.

Porges, S. W., McCabe, P. M., & Yongue, B. G. (1982). Respiratory-heart rate interactions: Psychological implications for pathophysiology and behavior. In J. J. Cacioppo & R. E. Petty (Eds.), *Perspectives in Cardiovascular Psychophysiology.* New York: Guilford.

Pujol R.,. & Hilding, D. (1973) Anatomy and physiology of the onset of auditory function. *Acta Otolaryyngologica, 76,* 1–10.

Querleu, D., & Renard, X. (1981) Bruit Intra-Uterin, Perceptions auditives et reactivate foetale aux stimulations sonores. *Medicine and Hygiene, 39,* 2102–2110.

Richards, J. E. (1985) Respiratory sinus arrhythmia predicts heart rate and isual responses during visual attention in 14 and 20 week old infants. *Psychophysiology, 22,* 101–109.

Rosner, B. and Doherty, N. (1971) The response of neonates to intra-uterine sounds. *Developmental Medicine and Child Neurology, 21,* 723–729.

Rubel, E. W. (1985) Auditory System Development. In G. Gottlieb & N. A. Krasnegor (Eds.), *Measurement of Audition and Vision in the First Year of Postnatal Life: A Methodological Overview.* Norwood, NJ: Ablex.

Satt, B. J. (1985) An investigation into the acoustical induction of intra-uterine learning, Ph. D. Dissertation, California of Professional Psychology.

Sontag, L. W., & Wallace, R. F. (1936) Changes in the rate of fetal heart in response to vibratory stimuli. *American Journal of Disabled Children*, *51*, 583−589.

Spence, M. J., & DeCasper, A. J. (1987) Prenatal experience with low-frequency maternal-voice sounds influence neonatal perception of maternal voice samples. *Infant Behavior and Development*, 10, 133−142.

Starr, A., Amlie, R. N., Martin, W. H. & Sanders, S. (1977) Development of auditory function in newborn infants revealed by auditory brainstem potentials, *Pediatrics*, *60*, 831−839.

Turkewitz, G. (in press) A prenatal source for the development of hemispheric specialization. In S. Segalowitz & D. Molfese (Eds.) *Developmental Implication of Brain Lateralization.*

Versyp, F. (1985) Transmission intra-amniotique des sons et des voix humanines, Thesis for doctoral degree in medicine, Univ. at Lille, France.

Vince, M. A., Billing, B. A., Baldwin, B. A., Toner, J. N., & Weller, C. (1985). Maternal vocalisations and other sound in the fetal lamb's sound environment. *Early Human Development*, 1985, *11*, 179−190.

Werker, J., Gilbert, J., Humphrey, K. & Tees, R. (1981) Developmental aspects of cross-language speech perception. *Child Development*, *52*, 349−355.

Zajonc, R. B. (1980) Feeling and thinking. *American Psychologist*, *35*, 151−175.

Zajonc, R. B. (1984) On the primacy of affect. *American Psychologist*, *39*, 117−123.

PRENATAL–POSTNATAL CONTINUITY

Embryonic Motor Output and Movement Patterns: Relationship to Postnatal Behavior

Anne Bekoff

EPO Biology Dept.
University of Colorado
Boulder, Colorado

Even cursory observation of embryonic motor activity in any of a variety of species of birds or mammals is sufficient to convince the observer that this is a distinctive form of behavior. This, in turn, raises questions about its relationship to later behavior. To explore the relationship between embryonic and postnatal behavior, we need to develop terminology and methodology that can adequately deal with both. This has been difficult to do for a number of reasons. One important contribution to the differences in appearance of prenatal and postnatal behavior is that, at most stages, the embryo is many times smaller than the newborn. In addition, the size of the embryo changes throughout development.

The small size of the embryo may also create problems in terms of resolution of the movements, making it difficult to resolve and characterize individual movements. Using film or video records can help to some extent by allowing the movements to be viewed more than once, in slow motion or even frame-by-frame. Furthermore, viewing or recording the behavior through a microscope can help alleviate the problems due to small size.

It is not just the smaller size that makes comparisons between the embryo and the postnatal animal problematic. There are also significant changes in morphometry. For example, the proximal limb segments elongate earlier than more distal segments and the proportions between segments may change (e.g., Hinchliffe & Johnson, 1980). Thus, movements that are otherwise similar may appear to differ.

Additional problems result from the fact that embryonic and postnatal behaviors are quite different in appearance (Hamburger, 1963; Hamburger & Oppenheim, 1967). For example, embryonic movements are often small in amplitude. Combined with the fact that embryos themselves are small, this creates further problems in resolution of the movements. In many cases the movements appear jerky. In contrast, movements occurring during most postnatal behavior appear relatively smooth. Furthermore, when more than one body part (e.g., hindlimb, forelimb, head) is active at the same time during embryonic behavior, the movements of the various body parts do not appear to be coordinated with one another. This lack of coordination contributes to the impression that the embryonic behavior is not "goal-oriented."

Another problem in the comparison of pre- and postnatal motor activity is that many of the postnatal behaviors that have been studied most extensively are rhythmical and repetitive (e.g., locomotion, feeding). Embryonic movements often occur periodically (see Robertson, this volume). However, within an activity period, the movements rarely appear rhythmical or repetitive. This irregularity makes them difficult to describe or to characterize.

BACKGROUND: METHODS AND TERMINOLOGY UNIQUE TO THE STUDY OF EMBRYONIC BEHAVIOR

Because embryonic behavior appears so distinctly different from most later behaviors, the terminology that has been developed to describe it is also distinctive. For example, many studies distinguish three categories of movement based on how much of the body is involved: (a) *total*, generalized mass movements; (b) *regional*, movements limited to the anterior or posterior part of the embryo; and (c) *local*, movements restricted to an individual part such as head, mouth or single limb (e.g., Angulo y Gonzalez, 1932; Barcroft & Barron, 1939; Narayanan, Fox & Hamburger, 1971; Windle & Griffin, 1931; Windle, Minear, Austin & Orr, 1935). A second way to describe the movements is to record the number of movements involving each of the various body parts, such as head, mouth, forelimbs, hindlimbs and trunk (Hamburger & Oppenheim, 1967; Oppenheim & Narayanan, 1968; Smotherman, Richards & Robinson, 1984). Additional categories can then be derived from these. For example, in addition to movements of individual body parts, *complex activity*, or the number of times 2 or more of the individual movements occur simultaneously, can be counted (see also Robinson & Smotherman, this volume).

A third approach is to distinguish three types of movements based on the form of the movements. For example, in their studies of chick embryos, Hamburger and his colleagues (Hamburger, 1963; Hamburger & Oppenheim, 1967) recognized one category, which they called Type I motility. During this type of embryonic behavior, the movements are relatively small in amplitude, jerky, and irregular. Furthermore, although various body parts may move simultaneously, coordination between body parts is not apparent. Type II motility consists of startles or sudden, rapid wriggles. Type III motility includes embryonic behaviors in which the movements are smoother and more coordinated in appearance than either Type I or II.

Type III motility is the most similar to later behavior. It is rhythmic and repetitive. In addition, it is "goal-oriented." For example, in chick embryos, Type III motility includes prehatching behaviors such as tucking, in which the head is moved into the hatching position and tucked underneath the right wing. Another Type III behavior is hatching itself. During hatching, smooth, coordinated movements are performed to crack the shell open so that the chick can escape at the end of incubation (Bakhuis, 1974; Bekoff & Kauer, 1984; Hamburger & Oppenheim, 1967; Kovach, 1970; Oppenheim, 1973).

Each of the methods mentioned above provides a very useful description of the embryonic movements. However, when the goal is to compare embryonic motility to later behaviors in order to elucidate possible relationships between them, additional methods are needed (see also Fentress & McLeod, this volume). The categories that have been developed for describing embryonic motility are not useful in describing postnatal behaviors. In fact, the unique terminology used to describe the embryonic movements emphasizes their distinctiveness and implies that there is no continuity with later behaviors.

Alternative Methods: EMG Recordings and Joint Angle Analysis

For comparing embryonic and postnatal behaviors, methods and terminology are needed that can be applied to both. Two methods have been used extensively to characterize a wide variety of rhythmic, repetitive postnatal behaviors in many different animals: electromyographic (EMG) recordings and joint angle measurements (for review, see Loeb & Gans, 1986). These 2 methods provide different kinds of information and are particularly powerful when used in combination. EMG recordings are typically made by inserting small wire electrodes into individual, identified muscles. The electrode leads are connected to the recording apparatus in such a way that the wires do not interfere with free movement of the subject. Recordings are then made while the animal performs the behavior of interest (Figure 1). Bursts of action potentials are seen each time an implanted muscle contracts. EMG recordings provide information about the pattern of muscle contractions that is involved in producing a set of

A. EMBRYONIC MOTILITY

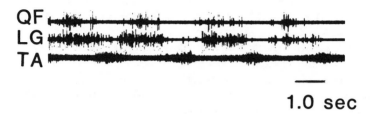

QF
LG
TA

1.0 sec

B. HATCHING

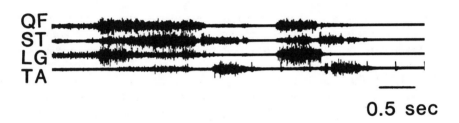

QF
ST
LG
TA

0.5 sec

C. WALKING

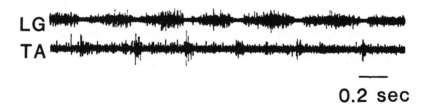

LG
TA

0.2 sec

Figure 1. EMG records show that a characteristic sequence of bursts is recorded from muscles of the right leg of the chick during each of three different behaviors. (A) Type I embryonic motility recorded from a 9-day old embryo. (B) Hatching recorded from a 21-day embryo. (C) Walking recorded from a 1-day old posthatching chick. Note the different time scales. ST = semitendinosus, a hip extensor and weak knee flexor; QF = quadriceps femoris, a knee extensor; LG = lateral gastrocnemius, an ankle extensor; TA = tibialis anterior, an ankle flexor.

movements. Thus, they provide an indirect measure of the *motor output* of the nervous system.

There are some technical problems that must be addressed in making EMG recordings from embryos. For example, as in making recordings from adults, care must be taken to ensure that there is not any cross-talk. That is, it is important to confirm that each electrode picks up activity from only one muscle, or, in some cases, from one compartment of a multifunctional muscle. The small size of embryos and the relative immaturity of the muscles may require the use of special electrodes. In the case of chick embryos, it has been possible to develop flexible electrodes that do not damage the delicate muscle tissue and do not restrict embryonic movements (Bekoff, 1976; Bekoff, Stein & Hamburger, 1975). Using these techniques, EMG recordings can be made from individual, identified muscles and the pattern of motor output produced by the embryonic nervous system can be compared to that produced during any one of a variety of later behaviors (Figure 1).

Quantitative analysis of EMG data can be used to identify similarities and/or differences between motor output patterns. For example, parameters such as the relative timing of activity in different muscles (phase values), the duration of EMG bursts in each muscle (burst durations) and the frequency with which each muscle is activated (cycle period) can be measured or calculated. When similarities are found in the EMG patterns recorded during different behaviors, they are often seen as suggesting that the same, or elements of the same, neural pattern generating circuitry is used (e.g., Bekoff, 1986; Bekoff, Nusbaum, Sabichi & Clifford, 1987). This kind of evidence is directly applicable to the issue of continuity between embryonic and postnatal behaviors.

Note, however, that the actual movements that are performed during a behavior cannot always be predicted based solely on EMG data. This is because the movements are a result of an interaction between the forces generated by the contraction of many muscles as well as a variety of other factors, such as initial position, inertia and musculoskeletal characteristics. To examine the actual movements, joint angle analysis, which is a form of kinematic, or movement, analysis can be used.

To carry out this type of analysis, certain points of interest on the surface of a subject (such as the joint of a limb) are marked to enhance their visibility. Next, the performance of a particular behavior is recorded on film or videotape. The points are then digitized to enter their x, y coordinates into a computer. From these coordinates, various parameters of the movements, such as joint angles, are calculated. These data can be analyzed and plotted in a variety of ways to allow quantitative assessment

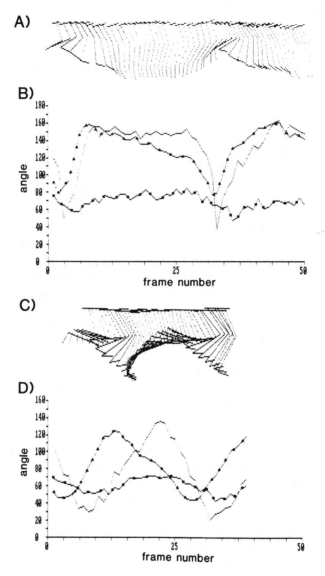

Figure 2. Comparison of kinematic data for the movements of the right leg of 2-day old posthatching chicks during consecutive frames of a walking sequence (A, B) and during consecutive frames of a swimming sequence (C, D). One frame = 16.7 msec. A) and C) each show stick figures plotted from digitized data. B) and D) each show hip (squares), knee (triangles) and ankle (line) angles (in degrees) plotted against frame number. Raw, unsmoothed, data have been plotted. Increasing angle represents extension, while decreasing angle represents flexion. Note that although the stick figures and graphs for the two behaviors are plotted on similar scales clear differences can be identified. (Based on data from Johnston & Bekoff, 1987).

of the movements (Figure 2). Thus, this kind of analysis provides information about the form of the movements that are performed. Furthermore, joint angle analysis allows quantitative comparison of movements in animals of different sizes and/or morphometry and comparison of different behaviors.

Thus, EMG recordings and joint angle analysis provide ways of quantifying motor output and movement patterns, respectively. Furthermore, by using time marks placed simultaneously on both EMG and film or video records, it is possible to correlate the motor output with the movements. As will be seen in the following section, these techniques are particularly useful in the context of comparing behaviors that are very different in appearance.

WHAT HAVE WE LEARNED ABOUT PRENATAL-POSTNATAL CONTINUITY FROM EMG AND KINEMATIC RECORDINGS?

EMG recordings have been used to examine the development of reflex responses in guinea pig and sheep embryos (Anggard, Bergstrom & Bernhard, 1961; Bergstrom, Hellstrom & Stenberg, 1962). However, this technique has been applied to the study of normal, spontaneous embryonic behavior only in chick embryos (Bekoff, 1976; Bekoff, et al., 1975; Landmesser & O'Donovan, 1984). Chick embryos offer several advantages for this type of study. For example, fertile eggs are available throughout the year. In addition, the embryos are easily accessible at all stages of the 20 to 21 day incubation period. A hole can be made in the shell through which the embryo can be observed and manipulated. Thus the embryo can be maintained in its normal environment during recording sessions. A further advantage is that because each embryo is encased in its own eggshell, it can be maintained apart from the mother as long as appropriate conditions of heat and humidity are supplied. There is no placental connection to consider as there is in mammals.

Analyses of EMG recordings from leg muscles in chick embryos have shown that, despite the uncoordinated appearance of the Type I embryonic movements, the nervous system produces a coordinated pattern of muscle contraction (Figure 1; Bekoff, 1976; Bekoff, et al., 1975; Bradley & Bekoff, 1987; Landmesser & O'Donovan, 1984). That is, within a leg, antagonist muscles are active in alternation, while synergists are coactive. In addition, coordination of muscles of the two legs, or interlimb coordination, is also seen (Cooper, 1983). Furthermore, this coordinated pattern of leg motor output is seen at the time the earliest leg movements occur at 6 to 7 days of incubation (Bekoff, et al., 1975; Cooper, 1983; O'Donovan, 1987). This is before the first cutaneous reflex arcs become functional, which is not until 7.5 to 8 days of incubation (Narayanan & Malloy, 1974; Oppenheim, 1972; Visintini & Levi-Montalcini, 1939). Therefore the neural circuitry underlying the production of these coordinated movements is established in the absence of sensory input.

Previous work suggests that there is continuity between the motor output patterns seen during embryonic motility and the patterns seen during hatching and walking (Bekoff, 1976; 1986). Despite the fact that there are large, obvious differences among the EMG patterns seen during these three behaviors, there are also some similarities. As can be seen in Figure 1, the basic pattern of muscle activation is similar in all three behaviors. That is, muscles that are coactive in one behavior tend to be coactive in the others. Similarly, those muscles that alternate in one behavior also alternate in the others. For example, gastrocnemius (LG) and tibialis (TA) alternate in embryonic motility, hatching and walking. Thus, although there are substantial differences in the motor output patterns, there are also similarities that suggest the possibility that neural circuitry is conserved and re-used in different behaviors.

Another indication of continuity is provided by the observation that there is a gradual transition in some features of the pattern from Type I motility at 17 days to hatching on day 20 or 21 (Figure 3). In contrast to the gradual transition that can be seen in some aspects of the leg motor output patterns of Type I motility and hatching, an abrupt transition is seen from hatching to walking. Walking begins within a few hours after the chick completes hatching (Vince & Chinn, 1972). Once the chick escapes from the shell, hatching behavior ceases and is not normally initiated again. Nevertheless, recent work has shown that the hatching leg motor output can be re-elicited from a posthatching chick if it is placed in the hatching position in an artificial egg (Bekoff & Kauer, 1984). Hatching can be elicited at least as late as 61 days posthatching, the age of the oldest chicks tested. Thus the circuitry for hatching remains functional in the posthatching chick. This means that it co-exists in time with the circuitry for walking. Furthermore, this result eliminates the possibility that the hatching circuitry is either dismantled or permanently modified to produce the walking circuitry.

Evidence that the neural circuitry used for the production of the leg movements of hatching is re-used to produce walking is provided by a recent study in which hatching and walking in normal and deafferented chicks are compared (Bekoff et al., 1987). In this study, analysis of EMG recordings showed that several of the differences seen between the leg motor output patterns of hatching and walking were decreased or eliminated by removing sensory input from the legs. Thus, the walking leg motor output pattern becomes more similar to the pattern seen during hatching.

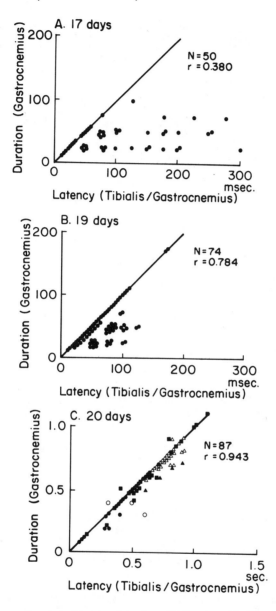

Figure 3. Latency-duration plots showing when tibialis, an ankle flexor, becomes active relative to the time of termination of activity in gastrocnemius, an ankle extensor. Data are shown for embryonic motility in 17-day (A) and 19-day (B) chick embryos and for hatching in 20-day embryos (C). Clustering of points near the 45° diagonal line and high correlation coefficients (r) indicate tight coupling between the termination of gastrocnemius and onset of tibialis bursts. Scatter of points and low correlation coefficients indicate less tight coupling. Note the gradual increase in coupling from 17 to 20 days of incubation. (From Bekoff, 1981).

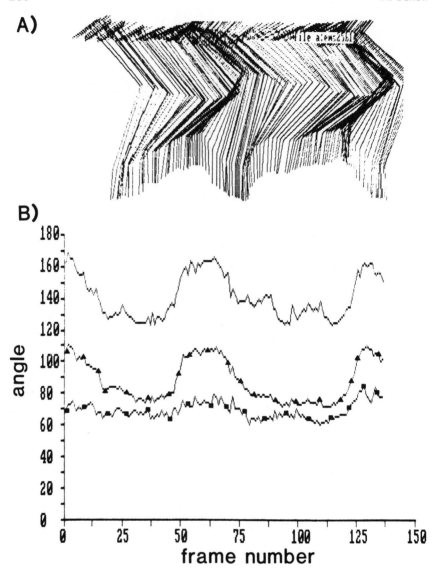

Figure 4. Kinematic data for the right leg of a 10-day old chick embryo during Type I motility. Data are derived from consecutive frames of a sequence of movements in which coordination of hip, knee and ankle is seen. One frame = 16.7 msec. A) Stick figures plotted from digitized data. B) Joint angles (in degrees) of hip (square), knee (triangles) and ankle (line) plotted against frame number. Raw, unsmoothed, data have been plotted. Note that all three joints extend (increasing angle) and flex (decreasing angle) together. (Based on data from Watson & Bekoff, 1987.)

These results are consistent with the hypothesis that sensory input from the legs normally modulates the output of a single pattern generating circuit to produce the two different leg motor patterns of hatching and walking.

Therefore, analysis of EMG data from embryonic motility, hatching and walking in chicks supports the idea that there is prenatal-postnatal continuity at the level of neural pattern generating circuitry. How can this be reconciled with the clear discontinuities that have been seen at the behavioral level? We do not yet have the complete answer to this question. However, work currently being done on the kinematics of embryonic motility in chicks is providing some clues (Watson & Bekoff, 1987). Joint angle data from 9- and 10-day old embryos have shown that coordination is present between hip, knee and ankle in many embryonic leg movements (Figure 4). Furthermore, coordination between left and right legs can also be observed in some movement sequences (S. J. Watson, personal communication). Nevertheless, aspects of the embryonic leg movements such as cycle period, amplitude and initial direction of leg movement (extension or flexion) vary widely. Kinematic patterns seen in chick embryos and those seen using the same techniques in posthatching chicks are currently being compared to gain further understanding of why the behaviors appear so different.

QUESTIONS FOR FUTURE RESEARCH

The studies discussed above suggest that, at least at some levels, there is continuity between embryonic and later behavior. Despite the clear differences in appearance of the behaviors, the neural circuitry underlying embryonic leg movements in chicks appears to be re-used to produce hatching at the end of the embryonic period and walking after hatching has been completed. However, one question that remains with regard to this finding is what accounts for the fact that embryonic behavior is so different in appearance from later behavior. As mentioned above, studies of the kinematics of chick embryonic motility should shed more light on this issue.

Behavioral observations have suggested that Type I motility in chick embryos appears similar throughout the incubation period. Thus, in the past, it has been considered to be a homogeneous behavior. Nevertheless, EMG records show that the underlying neural circuitry produces a variety of patterns of leg motor output (Figure 5; Bekoff, 1976). Therefore, it is relatively easy to look at an EMG record and determine the age of the embryo from which it was recorded. Neither the mechanisms by which

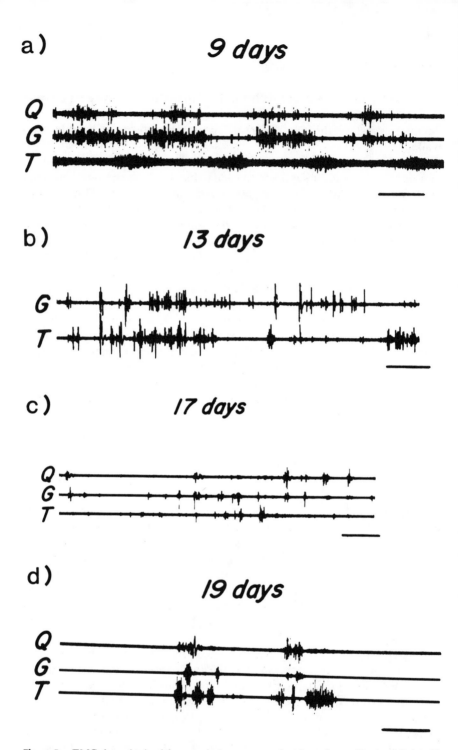

Figure 5. EMG data obtained from typical sequences of embryonic motility in a) 9-day, b) 13-day, c) 17-day and d) 19-day embryos. Time bar represents 1 sec in (a) and 500 msec in (b), (c) and (d). Note that distinctively different patterns are produced at each age. Q = quadriceps femoris, a knee extensor; G = lateral gastrocnemius, an ankle extensor; T = tibialis anterior, an ankle flexor. (Modified from Bekoff, 1976).

these diverse patterns are produced nor their significance is known. Furthermore, it will be interesting to carry out more detailed examination of the kinematics of the limb movements at different embryonic ages to determine whether there are, in fact, behavioral differences that can be identified and correlated with the differences seen in the EMG records.

In addition to the diversity of leg motor output patterns seen in embryos, there is obviously a diversity of patterns produced postnatally. For example, a postnatal animal may use its legs in walking, hopping, scratching or shaking to remove an irritant from the foot. One issue to be dealt with in the future is, then, to which postnatal behavior should the embryonic patterns be compared? Most commonly, the focus has been on determining whether continuity can be established between leg movements in the embryo and walking in the postnatal animal (Bekoff, 1986; Bekoff & Lau, 1980; Brown, 1915; Windle & Griffin, 1931). This is based on the reasonable assumption that walking is one of the most basic patterns of limb movement produced by the postnatal animal. Nevertheless, until further information becomes available, it may not be advisable to exclude other postnatal behaviors from consideration.

Another issue that remains to be addressed is that of how the movements of individual body parts are assembled into complete behaviors (see also Robinson & Smotherman, this volume). For example, most behavioral observations suggest that lack of coordination between body parts is one of the salient characteristics of embryonic motility in chicks (Hamburger, 1963; Hamburger and Oppenheim, 1967). One study has suggested that the wings become increasingly likely to be active simultaneously as embryonic development proceeds, while the right leg becomes less likely to be activated simultaneously with the wings (Provine, 1980). However, this study did not determine whether, during the simultaneous movements, the legs or wings were activated alternately or synchronously.

In the one available EMG study of interlimb coordination in chicks, both synchronous and alternating patterns of coordination were seen in the legs of the youngest embryos (7 days), while alternation alone was commonly seen later, at 8–11 days (Cooper, 1983). Kinematic studies currently underway have found both patterns in 9- to 10-day old chick embryos (Watson, unpublished data). No studies have yet examined coordination between the legs at later stages, between the wings, or between legs and wings, at any stage.

Interlimb coordination has been examined using film and videotape records of rat fetuses and in newborn rats during swimming (Bekoff & Lau, 1980; Bekoff & Trainer, 1979; Fentress, 1972). These studies show a gradual increase in the coordination among the four legs from late fetal to early postnatal life. Further analysis of coordination among body parts, including interlimb coordination, is likely to provide fertile ground for future studies.

At a behavioral level, the transitions from prenatal (embryonic motility) to perinatal (hatching) to postnatal (walking) behaviors are quite abrupt in the chick. However, there is reason to believe that there is continuity at the level of the underlying neural circuitry. That is, it appears that the circuitry used to generate the leg movements of embryonic motility is used later to produce the leg movements of hatching and that the circuitry, or elements of it, is also used to produce walking. Nevertheless, the available data only touch the surface in terms of understanding the relationship between embryonic and postnatal behaviors. Many interesting and challenging questions remain to be answered.

Acknowledgements

I would like to thank Dr. M. Bekoff, Dr. N. S. Bradley, R. M. Johnston and S. J. Watson for helpful comments on an earlier version of this manuscript. Some of the work presented here was supported by NSF grant BNS 79–13826 and NIH grant NS 20310.

References

Anggard, L., Bergstrom, R., & Bernhard, C. G. (1961). Analysis of prenatal spinal reflex activity in sheep. *Acta Physiol. Scand., 53*, 128–136.

Angulo y Gonzalez, A. W. (1932). The prenatal development of behavior in the albino rat. *Journal of Comparative Neurology, 55*, 395–442.

Bakhuis, W. L. (1974). Observations on hatching movements in the chick (*Gallus domesticus*). *Journal of Comparative and Physiological Psychology, 87*, 997–1003.

Barcroft, J., & Barron, D. H. (1939). The development of behaviour in foetal sheep. *Journal of Comparative Neurology, 70*, 447–502.

Bekoff, A. (1976). Ontogeny of leg motor output in the chick embryo: a neural analysis. *Brain Research, 106*, 271–291.

Bekoff, A. (1981). Embryonic development of chick motor behaviour. *Trends in Neuroscience, 4*, 181–183.

Bekoff, A. (1986). Ontogeny of chicken motor behaviours: evidence for multi-use limb pattern generating circuitry. In S. Grillner, P. S. G. Stein, D. G. Stuart, H. Forssberg & R. M. Herman, (Eds.), *Neurobiology of vertebrate locomotion*, (pp. 433–453). Hampshire, England: Macmillan.

Bekoff, A., & Kauer, J. A. (1984). Neural control of hatching: fate of the pattern generator for the leg movements of hatching in post-hatching chicks. *Journal of Neuroscience, 4*, 2659–2666.

Bekoff, A., & Lau, B. (1980). Interlimb coordination in 20-day-old rat fetuses. *Journal of Experimental Zoology, 214*, 173–175.

Bekoff, A., Nusbaum, M. P., Sabichi, A. L., & Clifford, M. (1987). Neural control of limb coordination: comparison of hatching and walking motor output patterns in normal and deafferented chicks. *Journal of Neuroscience, 7*, 2320–2330.

Bekoff, A., Stein, P. S. G., & Hamburger, V. (1975). Coordinated motor output in the hindlimb of the 7-day chick embryo. *Proceedings of the National Academy of Science, USA, 72*, 1245–1248.

Bekoff, A., & Trainer, W. (1979). Development of interlimb coordination during swimming in postnatal rats. *Journal of Experimental Biology, 83*, 1–11.

Bergström, R. M., Hellström, P.-E., & Stenberg, D. (1962). Studies in reflex irradiation in the foetal guinea-pig. *Ann. Chir. Gynaecol. Fenn., 51*, 171–178.

Bradley, N. S., & Bekoff, A. (1987). Emergence of flexion and extension muscle synergies in the hindlimb of chick embryos. *Society for Neuroscience Abstracts, 13*, 1504.

Brown, T. G. (1915). On the activities of the central nervous system of the unborn foetus of the cat; with a discussion of the question whether progression (walking, etc.) is a "learnt" complex. *Journal of Physiology (London), 49*, 208–215.

Cooper, M. W. (1983). Development of interlimb coordination in the embryonic chick. Ph.D. thesis, Yale University, New Haven, Conn.

Fentress, J. C. (1972). Development and patterning of movement sequences in inbred mice. In J. Kiger, (Ed.), *The biology of behavior*, (pp. 83–132). Corvallis: Oregon State University Press.

Hamburger, V. (1963). Some aspects of the embryology of behavior. *Quarterly Review of Biology, 38*, 342–365.

Hamburger, V., & Oppenheim, R. (1967). Prehatching motility and hatching behavior in the chick. *Journal of Experimental Zoology, 166*, 171–204.

Hinchliffe, J. R., & Johnson, D. R. (1980). *The development of the vertebrate limb*. Oxford: Clarendon Press.

Johnston, R. M., & Bekoff, A. (1987). Kinematic analysis of walking, swimming and air-stepping in chicks. *Society for Neuroscience Abstracts, 13*, 356.

Kovach, J. K. (1970). Development and mechanisms of behavior in the chick embryo during the last five days of incubation. *Journal of Comparative and Physiological Psychology, 73*, 392–406.

Landmesser, L. T., & O'Donovan, M. J. (1984). Activation patterns of embryonic chick hind limb muscles recorded in ovo and in an isolated spinal cord preparation. *Journal of Physiology (London), 347*, 189–204.

Loeb, G. E., & Gans, C. (1986). *Electromyography for experimentalists*. Chicago: University of Chicago Press.

Narayanan, C. H., Fox, M. W., & Hamburger, V. (1971). Prenatal development of spontaneous and evoked activity in the rat. *Behaviour, 40*, 100–134.

Narayanan, C. H., & Malloy, R. B. (1974). Deafferentation studies on motor activity in the chick. I. Activity pattern of hindlimb. *Journal of Experimental Zoology, 189*: 163–176.

O'Donovan, M. J. (1987). Experimental analysis of motor development in the chick embryo. In S. Grillner, P. S. G. Stein, D. G. Stuart, H. Forssberg & R. M. Herman, (Eds.), *Neurobiology of vertebrate locomotion*, (pp. 415–431). Hampshire, England: Macmillan.

Oppenheim, R. (1972). An experimental investigation of the possible role of tactile and proprioceptive stimulation in certain aspects of embryonic behavior in the chick. *Developmental Psychobiology, 5*, 71–91.

Oppenheim, R. (1973). Prehatching and hatching behavior: a comparative consideration. In G. Gottlieb, (Ed.), *Behavioral embryology*, (pp. 163–244). New York: Academic Press.

Oppenheim, R., & Narayanan, C. H. (1968). Experimental studies on hatching behavior in the chick. I. Thoracic spinal gaps. *Journal of Experimental Zoology, 168*, 387–394.

Provine, R. R. (1980). Development of between-limb movement synchronization in the chick embryo. *Developmental Psychobiology, 13*, 151–163.

Smotherman, W. P., Richards, L. S., & Robinson, S. R. (1984). Techniques for observing fetal behavior in utero: a comparison of chemomyelotomy and spinal transection. *Developmental Psychobiology, 17*, 661–674.

Vince, M. A., & Chinn, S. (1972). Effects of external stimulation on the domestic chick's capacity to stand and walk. *British Journal of Psychology, 63*, 89–99.

Visintini, F., & Levi-Montalcini, R. (1939). Relazione tra differenziazione strutturale e funzionale dei centri e delle vie nervose nell' embryone di pollo. *Schweiz. Archiv. Neurol. Psychol., 43*, 1–45.

Watson, S. J., & Bekoff, A. (1987). A kinematic study of chick embryonic motility. *Society for Neuroscience Abstracts, 13*, 1504.

Windle, W. F., & Griffin, A. M. (1931). Observations on embryonic and fetal movements of the cat. *Journal of Comparative Neurology, 52*, 149–188.

Windle, W. F., Minear, W. L., Austin, M. F., & Orr, D. W. (1935). The origin and early development of somatic behavior in the albino rat. *Physiological Zoology, 8*, 156–175.

On the Nature of Developing Motor Systems and the Transition from Prenatal to Postnatal Life

Esther Thelen
Department of Psychology
Indiana University
Bloomington, Indiana

Even the most altricial newborn comes into the world able to perform some coordinated movements. In many species, of course, newborns are endowed with a full complement of motor functions. Questions of the prenatal origins of such movement have engaged biologists and psychologists for over a century, and the publication of this volume attests to the continued importance of the developmental issues surrounding prenatal and postnatal behavior. Are fetal movements functional? Do they have current utility, or do these movements anticipate postnatal actions? Or are fetal movements only epiphenomena of a developing nervous system? Is there continuity between motor actions *in utero* and postnatal activity.

In this essay, I present a scheme for understanding the nature of early movement patterns and their developmental origins and fates. In particular, I seek to explain how the spontaneous activities of the fetus, embryo and larva may be related to the developing motor actions in the postnatal period. Species vary enormously in their relative functional maturity at birth, the ecological demands made upon them, and their subsequent developmental course. Nonetheless, my assumption here is that the same general principles of motor organization and the same fundamental developmental processes underlie emergent motor function in all vertebrate species.

GENERAL CHARACTERISTICS OF EARLY MOTOR BEHAVIOR

The traditional and one commonly accepted approach to developing motor systems—clearly seen in the legacy of Coghill, McGraw, Hamburger, and others—is to relate emergent function to its material structure, the developing nervous system. It is undeniably true that nervous system development sets the absolute ceiling on behavior and that a full understanding of the ontogeny of behavior must include knowledge of these structure-function relations. But I also believe that the traditional approach in itself is not sufficient to explain emergent function. In particular, the strict neurogenic approach provides no principled explanation for five general characteristics of movement in the prenatal and early postnatal period. These include (a) the spontaneity of early movement, (b) its cyclicity or rhythmicity, (c) the degree of coordination, (d) the lack of one-to-one correspondence between neural activity and behavior, and (e) its context specificity. I suggest here that a view of motor development based on dynamic principles of complex systems may be more successful in addressing these puzzles as animals make the transition between prenatal and postnatal life.

A number of comprehensive recent reviews (e.g., Bekoff, 1981; Fentress & McLeod, 1986; Hall & Oppenheim, 1987; Prechtl, 1981; Provine, 1986; Smotherman & Robinson, 1988) document the nearly bewildering array of species-specific early motor patterns and behavioral adaptations. Despite this variability, several common themes emerge. First is that all embryos, fetuses, larvae, and newborn vertebrates become spontaneously active at some point in their gestation (see Bekoff; Provine, this volume). Spontaneous means that movements of limb and body segments, activation of muscle groups, or movement-related activity in the central nervous system can be detected in the absence of specific or identifiable eliciting stimuli. Hall and Oppenheim (1987, p. 96) have called such spontaneous behavior "a primary and fundamental feature of the earliest stages of ontogeny".

Embryonic, fetal and newborn movements are, in addition, very often rhythmical or cyclical in their organization. Cycle periods range widely from the seconds or fractions of seconds of the microstructure of sucking and kicking, the seconds or minutes of rhythms of spontaneous motility seen in embryos, older fetuses, and newborns (e.g. Robertson, Dierker, Sorokin, & Rosen, 1982; see also Robertson, this volume) the ultradian rhythms (40–90 minutes) characteristic of sleep/wake cycles in mammalian fetuses and newborns, and the circadian cycles of rest and activity usually acquired after birth (see Reppert & Weaver, this volume). At birth, for example, the human newborn has several layers of embedded rhythmicities: repetitive kicking embedded within periods of spontaneous motility and quiescence embedded within cyclic changes of behavioral state.

Within this rhythmic superstructure, movement in the prenatal and perinatal period may show coordination of varying degrees from tightly patterned to random or disorganized. We can define a movement as patterned or coordinated if the limbs or body segments move, or muscle segments contract, in a nonrandom fashion with respect to one another in time or in space; that is, muscles and segments act synergistically rather than as isolated units. By this definition, the so-called "mass movements" seen in avian and mammalian embryos would appear to be uncoordinated: limbs, segments, and body parts flex and extend, twist, or open and close in disorganized fashion, with little predictable relations. Many early movements, however, appear to be highly organized, including tail oscillations, alternating and synchronous stepping, kicking or "swimming" movements, hatching, wing-flapping, respiratory movements, sucking, swallowing, grooming, startles, hand-face contacts, stretching, and defensive reflexes. In general, coordination increases with increasing gestational age.

Most importantly, however, there is often no one-to-one correspondence between activity measured at the neural level and the observed fetal or newborn behavior. That is, one cannot infer behavior directly from observing the events at the neural level, and conversely, one cannot predict the pattern of neural activity from the manifest behavior. Bekoff (1976), for example, discovered regularly alternating bursts of agonist/antagonist activity in ankle muscles of chick embryos (*Gallus gallus*) at 7 days, long before coordination in movement could be detected in the limb or the functional appropriation of that pattern for locomotion. Likewise, Stehouwer & Farel (1983) described patterned synaptic activation of hindlimb motorneurons in bullfrog tadpoles (*Rana catesbeiana*) at a stage before the limbs were morphologically well differentiated or ennervated. In newborn infants, in contrast, leg kicking movements were seemingly *more* complex in their time-space trajectories than their very simple, coactive muscle firing patterns would suggest (Thelen & Fisher, 1983). Indeed, when infants learn to walk independently, their EMG patterns retain many of these "primitive" characteristics, and only assume adult-like patterns over many months or years (Okamoto & Goto, 1985). Thus, we have a developmental paradox: in some cases, highly coordinated neural activity is not translated into equally coordinated movement (more is less), and in other cases, coordinated movement emerges from a seemingly less-organized neural basis (less is more).

Finally, although the underlying structural substrates for movement are necessarily paced by organic maturation, behavioral expression is essentially determined by the context of the organism. By manipulating the context, researchers have accelerated the performance of behaviors usually not seen until later ontogenetic stages or "restored" movements believed to be lost or inhibited. For example, Stehouwer and Farel (1984) promoted earlier use of the hindlimbs in bullfrog tadpoles by providing them with wet and dry solid substrates. Chicks flapped their poorly developed and featherless wings when dropped (Provine, 1981). In exteriorized rat fetuses, Robinson and Smotherman (1987) observed more synchronous movements when fetuses were viewed in the amniotic sac or a warm water bath than when they were confined within the uterus. Supporting newborn mice upright elicited complex grooming movements usually not performed until several days later (Fentress, 1981). When Hall (1979) provided rat pups with the right thermal environment and food, they ingested food independent of the mother long in advance of the normal appearance of this ability. And human infants, when supported over a motorized tread-mill, performed mature-like, coordinated, alternating stepping movements many months before they were able to walk independently (Thelen, 1986a).

Contextual manipulations can also "restore" behaviors believed to have "disappeared" from the movement repertoire of the developing animal. Chick embryos hatch, for example, by a series of well-coordinated, synchronous thrusting leg movements. Bekoff and Kauer (1984) elicited these characteristic hatching movements in chicks as much as 61 days post hatching by folding them into appropriately sized glass eggs. Although the hatching movements are usually never seen after normal hatching, the postural context of the chick—likely the position of the head—elicited this coordinated behavior (Bekoff & Kauer, 1982). Human infants nor-mally do not perform the so-called newborn stepping movements after about 2 months of age. However, the pattern could be restored by simple postural or contextual manipulations—in this case, by placing the infant supine or submerging the legs in water (Thelen & Fisher, 1982; Thelen, Fisher, & Ridley-Johnson, 1984). In each of these cases, then, the presumed availability of the patterned movement ability was not sufficient to ensure its performance. The animals appeared to be organized, not by their maturational status, per se, but also by the context or the tasks they faced. The role of context in organizing behavior may be equally important prenatally as postnatally (see Smotherman & Robinson, this volume).

PRINCIPLES OF COMPLEX, SELF-ORGANIZING SYSTEMS

How, then, can developing motor systems be characterized to account for the phenomena of spontaneity, cyclicity, coordination, nonequivalence, and context-specificity? Central nervous system events alone cannot be the causal agents of movement or developmental change because the CNS may either overspecify or underspecify behavior. Instead, I rely on a more general dynamic systems view of motor organization and develop-mental change. The basic assumption of this view is that moving and developing organisms are multicomponent systems that obey the same principles as other complex physical, chemical, and biological systems composed of many cooperating elements. There currently is much interest in how such complex systems can generate ordered behavior or spatio-temporal patterning. In dynamical terms, the question may be phrased to ask how a physical or biological system composed of many elements can produce behavior that can be described by far fewer variables than the cooperating elements.

The application of the principles emerging from this field of nonlinear dynamical systems to biological systems is in its infancy, but holds much promise for modeling phenomena in neurobiology, physiology, neural network behavior, and motor and perceptual systems (Haken, 1983, 1985; Kelso & Schöner, in press; Nicolis, 1986). Note here that Kelso and his colleagues have provided rigorous confirmation of the dynamical organization of movement with mathematical modeling of adult rhythmical hand and speech movements (e.g. Kelso & Scholz, in press; Kelso, Scholz, & Schöner, 1986; Schöner, Haken, & Kelso, 1986). Such a mapping from observations to theory has not yet been accomplished with a developmental phenomenon (and may be a difficult or even impossible feat with such inherently noisy and nonstationary systems). Nonetheless, the principles may provide an equally fruitful approach to the study of early behavioral development (see also, Fentress, 1986; Fogel & Thelen, 1987; Kugler, Kelso, & Turvey, 1982; Thelen & Fogel, in press; Thelen, Kelso, & Fogel, 1987; Wolff, 1986), and especially, may offer new paradigms for uniting research and modeling to understand emerging coordination within the matrix of both stability and change.

I present here, in abbreviated form, a characterization of moving and developing organisms consistent with dynamical principles (Thelen, Kelso, & Fogel, 1987).

(1) Moving and developing organisms are complex biological systems composed of the cooperative interactions of many subsystems and processes, and composed of many material substrates operating on different time scales.

(2) It is the nature of such complex systems to produce ordered and patterned behavior that can be described with far fewer variables than those that compose the ensemble. Imagine, for example, humans performing simple motor actions like reaching or walking. A nearly infinite number of anatomical elements and physiological processes must act in cooperation to produce these behaviors. Yet the behaviors themselves may be completely described by relatively few kinematic and kinetic variables specifying trajectories, limb phase relations, or output forces over time. At whatever level of behavioral description, these parameters act to compress the original high number of degrees of freedom inherent in the system to a description of much lower dimensionality. In dynamical

systems terminology, parameters which compress information are called order parameters.

In complex systems, this cooperative effect—the compression of the degrees of freedom to produce ordered space-time behavior—is strictly an autonomous and self-organizing phenomenon. That is, order is a function of the systems interactions of the components in a particular context. There need be no higher order set of instructions either inside or outside the system prescribing the resulting pattern. In our motor example, then, we presume that no specific and iconic representations of walking or reaching need exist in the organism before the execution of the act. The order exists only as the system assembles to perform the action under certain task and energy constraints.

Self-organization is common in many physical systems. We do not expect genetic or neural codes prescribing intricate crystal patterns, laser light formations, cloud layers, and so on. Likewise, the increase of complexity in developing systems is emergent from the cooperativity of the ensemble, not from prescriptive codes existing before the ontogenetic course unfolds (see Oyama, 1985).

(3) Let us imagine, then, plotting the behavior of an organism as a function of the order parameters. In our movement example, we might choose two variables, the position and the velocity of the limb, that would completely describe its behavior in time and space. If the behavior is not random, this behavior trajectory is confined to a particular region of the plot and shows a particular ordered topology. In Figure 1, Carolyn Heriza (1986) has constructed such a plot for the angular excursions of the knee joint in leg kicking movements in two premature infants, which is quite rhythmical and coordinated. When the behavior of an infant's knees is plotted as a function of its position and velocity, it occupies only a particular region on the state space defined by those parameters.

Such coordinated behaviors that are stationary and reproducible over the period of observation can be considered as stable attractor states of the order parameter dynamics (Kelso & Schöner, in press). In dynamical formulations, attractors are preferred regions of the abstract state space, that is, regions where the time-space trajectories of the behavior tend to converge (see Abraham & Shaw, 1982). (In contrast, trajectories of random behavior would not occupy any preferred regions of the abstract state space.) Behaviors may, in turn, exhibit different attractor regimes: a single, reproducible limb movement, for example, may be characterized by a point attractor regime. Repetitive, cyclical behaviors, of special interest in early development, are characterized as periodic attractors, as illustrated in Figure 1. The presence of periodic attractors indicates that

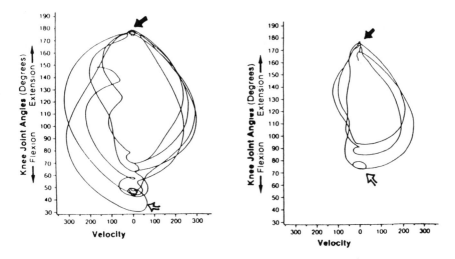

Figure 1. Phase plane trajectories of angular rotations of the knee joint during 10 sec of spontaneous rhythmical kicking movements, by a premature infant at 34 weeks gestational age (left panel) and the same infant at 40 weeks. The phase plane plots the movement amplitude (angles of flexion and extension) versus its instantaneous velocity, and is a depiction of the dynamical behavior of the system in a state space. Time is not explicitly represented. What is noteworthy is the resemblance to the classical periodic attractor in dynamics (see Abraham & Shaw, 1982), indicating an underlying topological stability, which is, in turn, similar to the dynamic stability exhibited by other mature rhythmic behaviors such as speech (see Thelen, Kelso, & Fogel, 1987). From Heriza (1986).

the system tends to remain in a stable cyclical orbit despite transient perturbations; it is a perferred mode of motion for the system under certain conditions.

(4) Behavioral patterns can change from one attractor regime to another. Since the behavior is a function of both the organism and the task or context, variables or parameters both intrinsic to the organism and external to it may modify the behavioral patterns, or shift the system into new stable states.

(5) At points of transition, a control parameter is the internal or external parameter (one or several of the many possible component variables) that shifts the system into a new dynamic regime. The control parameter may be rather unspecific and is not a prescriptive instruction for change. In dynamical systems, then, small quantitative changes in only one component or in the context may be amplified to produce

qualitative shifts in the outcome behavior. In infant leg kicking, for example, as the infant becomes quiet—a quantitative change in behavioral arousal—it will shift from a kicking to a non-kicking mode—a qualitative change in behavior (Thelen, Kelso, & Fogel, 1987).

(6) In developing systems, new behavior patterns may arise from two processes (Fogel & Thelen, 1987): (a) There may be underlying scalar change in the control parameter. For example, changes in a component resulting from growth may serve to shift the entire organism into a new behavioral mode. (b) The nature of the control parameters may themselves change over time and in different contexts. This means that the elements that shift the system into new forms themselves are nonstationary, a reflection of the asynchronous and nonlinear nature of development of the components of the developing system and its changing environmental demands and niches.

A SYSTEMS CHARACTERIZATION OF EARLY MOTOR DEVELOPMENT

I now use these abstract principles to characterize developing motor systems and especially their spontaneity, cyclicity, coordination, non-equivalence and context-specificity. Embryos, fetuses, larvae, and newborn animals are, as are all biological organisms, multicomponent systems with anatomical structures and physiological processes cooperating to produce behavior. At any point in time, the behavior of the organism is a function of the biological constraints of that maturational stage and the task or context of the animal.

Spontaneity of movement, therefore, need not be evidence of "design," but is rather the natural, autonomous output of a particular configuration of anatomical units and physiological processes under certain energy constraints. This is not to say that spontaneous movements are without function, but that function is not an essential precursor to spontaneity, as spontaneity may arise *de novo* and without phylogenetic prescription. Whether normal function depends on the exercise of prenatal or perinatal movements is left as an empirical question. For example, suppression of neurological activity in amphibian embryos does not impair eventual swimming (Haverkamp, 1986; Haverkamp & Oppenheim, 1986), but similar narcosis will lead to abnormal development in chick embryos (Oppenheim, Pittman, Gray & Maderdrut, 1978). Yet even with no apparent selective pressures to move, animal embryos do so spontaneously because of their emergent organization. Functional appropriation of those movements would be a secondary ontogenetic adaptation. Although alternating leg movements may serve to rotate the human fetus, which may indeed have benefits (Prechtl, 1986), one cannot presume that either the coordinative pattern or its spontaneous activation are specific ontogenetic adaptations for this purpose.

I make a similar claim for the phenomenon of cyclicity. Many natural systems are cyclical; Kugler, Kelso, & Turvey (1980) argue compellingly that assemblies of muscles in the neuromotor system use energy in the particular fashion of dissipative structures. That is, they draw energy from the underlying metabolic processes in "squirts", which lead naturally to oscillations. The periodicity of the oscillations arise, however, not from any inherent "clock" functions. "The 'timing' of impulses does not require a separate device but arises necessarily from the design specifications—the equations of constraint—of the muscle collective" (p. 18). Thus, we may explain the nested levels of cyclicity as a function of the particular collectives involved and might predict a different period of oscillation for wholebody "mass" movements, for example, than for single limbs or body segments. The characterization of muscle collectives as autonomous oscillators thereby raises the possibility of von Holst-like relations among oscillators—phenomena of coupling and entrainment. Contemporary theorists have demonstrated how such constellations of oscillators can produce behavior of remarkable complexity and flexibility. Again, we need not invoke either ontogenetic or phylogenetic design to this patterning, although the regularity may *a posteriori* provide the organism with some functional benefit (see Robertson, this volume).

What about coordination? In this dynamic view, coordination is not a consequence of "hard-wired" neural elements, but rather a "soft-assembly" or preferential linkage of elements in response to context or task. Emergent coordination can be envisioned, therefore, as progressively more stable preferential linkages or attractor regimes. The phylogenetic history of the species as expressed through its anatomical and neurological structure sets the ultimate limits on these preferential energy configurations, but within those constraints, the immediate context or task recruits the output pattern. This means that a pattern that is stable under one circumstance may not be stable under other conditions, even when the maturational status of the organism is similar. The control parameters that shift the system into new stable attractor regimes thus may be intrinsic to the organism, as scalar changes in growth, or extrinsic, in the context. For example, Robinson and Smotherman (1987; this volume) have described the emergence of synchronous movements in the rat fetus as increasingly more likely associations between adjacent body regions, suggesting that certain assemblies of muscle groups became more stable with age. However, within a maturational stage, context was also a determining factor, as rats exhibited more complex movements when exteriorized from the restraining fetal membranes and observed in a bath.

The fluid assembly of coordinative patterns thus allows both context-specificity and nonequivalence. For example, rhythmic alternation of lower limb muscle collectives appears to be a stable property of many vertebrate systems, ranging from agonist/antagonist activity in early chick embryos to cyclic leg actions in rat fetuses and in human fetuses and newborns. We might speculate that this preferential pattern is a result of the necessity for limbed vertebrates to produce alternations for locomotion. Nonetheless, the expression of these patterns both pre- and postnatally, i.e., their stability, is entirely dependent on a facilitative context, which includes the necessary biomechanical conditions. In both chicks and frog larvae, for example, neurogenic alternations can be detected long in advance of their behavioral expressions. In rats and humans, manipulations of the biomechanical constraints—posture, limb masses, or the supportive medium—can elicit or suppress alternating limb movements. Similarly, if it is the context which organizes the behavior, organisms may not be bound to a one-on-one, fixed solution to task demands. The stability of the output behavior is independent of the particular material structures or muscle combinations that produce it. Berkenblit, Feldman, and Fukson (1986) provide a dramatic example of this phenomena (also referred to as motor equivalence). When an irritant was placed on the back of a spinal frog, the frog's hind limbs performed accurate wiping movements to the source of irritation regardless of the initial position of the limb. Clearly, completely different muscle actions were needed to move the leg depending on the initial position. Yet even in this simple preparation, the task organized the movement. Similar task-specificity is apparent in the so-called reflexes of early human newborn, such as hand-to-mouth behavior, rooting, sucking, and wiping reactions, as well as in the adjustments in arm and leg actions seen after the newborn period.

IMPLICATIONS FOR THE PRE- TO POSTNATAL TRANSITION

A dynamic perspective leads to several important implications for motor behavior and the transition from pre- to postnatal life. First, the uterus or egg is just as much an environment or context for action as the postnatal world, a point made eloquently by Smotherman and Robinson (1988). Although changes in the prenatal environment may be more modulated, the embryo's environment system profoundly affects the motor outcome. Studies in several species have documented, for example, that the restraints imposed on growing embryos by egg or uterine walls may restrict movement frequency or complexity (see Moessinger, this volume).

Within both the prenatal and postnatal context, organisms may display increasingly stable motor attractor regimes as the preferred coordinative modes become expressed. However, it is important to note that during ontogeny, the nature of the control parameters may change. At times, the control parameters for the performance of stable modes may be the neurological structure or the effector anatomy. That is, these organismic components may shift the animal into new output configurations. However, at other ontogenetic stages, aspects of the context may act as the control parameter. Indeed, as Oyama (1985) has pointed out, controls themselves emerge as a result of the hierarchical interactions of the components during ontogeny.

For terrestrial species, the transition from prenatal to postnatal life presents an abrupt change not only in the physiological and behavioral demands on the organism, but on the entire context for action, and we are not surprised to find major reorganization of behavior. While the continuity between the two life stages may be reflected in the establishment and maintenance of some preferred coordinative patterns, the demands of postnatal life shift the system into new and specific performance modes. The time course of the emergence of more adult-like actions would then be a function of the stability of the established preferred coordinations and the nature of the specific postnatal demands. In precocial species, the coordinative patterns for many adaptive actions must respond rapidly to task demands, while in altricial species this time course is relaxed, although certain coordinative modes, such as sucking in mammals, must be highly stable and reproducible immediately after birth.

CONTROL PARAMETERS IN THE PRE- TO POSTNATAL TRANSITION

Thus, an important empirical question is to determine the essential control parameters at this ontogenetic transition. What are the continuities between prenatal and postnatal life and what are the factors that shift the system into new forms of behavior? Here I look at the relation between this transition and several intriguing aspects of coordinated leg movements in three species: frog, chick, and human.

Frog

Stehouwer and Farel (1983; 1984; 1985) have elegantly documented the onset of hindlimb locomotor activity in the larval bull frog (tadpole). Tadpoles swim by undulating their tails, while after metamorphosis, frogs locomote by using their hindlimbs either alternately (stepping) or synchronously (frog kicking). As mentioned above, these investigators discovered activation of hindlimb motoneurons in patterns corresponding to stepping in tadpoles before the bones and muscles of the hindlimbs had differentiated or were ennervated, and kicking patterns developed soon thereafter.

Despite the early presence of the neural substrate for this behavior (Stage III), actual use of the hindlimbs showed a more complex course. When tadpoles were tested in deep water, first use of the hindlimbs appeared as simple bilateral extensions at Stages XII to XVI, followed by unilateral movements for correction and rolling (Stage XV) and bilateral movements to "take off" and "land" (Stages XIV to XIX). Hindlimb use increased dramatically after Stage XVII, when the use of the limbs for locomotion commenced. Concomitantly, use of the tail for locomotion decreased precipitously between Stages XXI and XXIII.

What, then, were the control parameters driving these distinct developmental phase shifts? Both behavioral and electrophysiological measures of the stability and reliability of the hindlimb coordinative pattern indicated gradual improvement from Stages XII to XXV, with none of the discontinuities seen in the actual performance pattern. More revealing were a series of clever contextual manipulations that indicated that the entire developmental course of hindlimb locomotor use was a function of the test context. When these authors tested the tadpoles on either a wet slippery surface or a dry hard surface rather than deep water, the tadpoles used their hindlimbs in preference to their tails for locomotion at considerably earlier stages; the dry surface shifted the transition to hindlimb use by as much as five developmenal stages (Figure 2).

The neurological substrate for hindlimb locomotion is clearly a necessary component, but not a sufficient cause for the behavioral performance. In a dynamic systems view, we can imagine that the coordinative patterns for stepping or hopping become increasingly stable with age, but that the relative stability is equally emergent from the context. With a minimum threshold of coordinative maturation, some, as yet unknown, aspects of the environment, act as control parameters to shift the tadpole into new ontogenetic forms. As Stehouwer and Farel (1984) point out, tadpoles naturally begin to prefer shallow places along the shore to deep water at Stage XX (metamorphosis commences at Stage XVIII). At the same time, the hindlimb movements only become effective for forward propulsion on land after this stage, when the forelimbs can provide postural support. The improvements in locomotor quality may be considered as context-driven. Since the basic neurological mechanisms are in place, the substrate affords the tadpole the opportunity to practice adjustments in force and orientation necessary for precise control of the behavior. No amount of

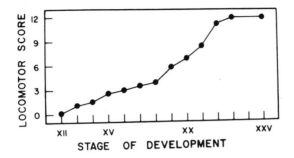

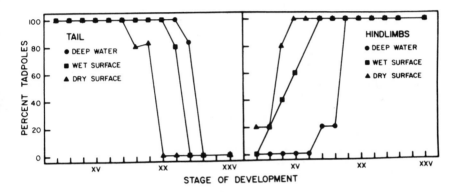

Figure 2. Context-dependent discontinuities in use of tail and hindlimbs in frog tadpoles. (A). Mean composite scores of locomotor maturity as a function of stage of development. Note the gradual maturation of locomotor abilities. (B). Percent of larvae using their tails (left panel) and hindlimbs (right panel) for locomotion as a function of test substrate. Note sharp discontinuities. (From Stehouwer & Farel, 1984; Reprinted by permission of John Wiley & Sons, copyright, 1984).

practice in deep water can anticipate the postural and biomechanical demands of terrestrial locomotion.

Chick

Hatching in chicks provides another illustration where the pre- to postnatal transition engenders several dramatic phase shifts in preferred limb coordinations. As in frog tadpoles, electrophysiological evidence of coordinated muscle activity can be detected in chick embryos long before the overt behavior appears organized. This temporal coupling of the muscle groups improves during development. Although elements of characteristic prehatching movements can be seen in the few days prior to hatching, hatching behavior itself begins rather abruptly on day 20. Hatching consists of highly stereotyped sequences of movements including strong thrusting movements of the legs. After hatching, these movements are typically not seen again, although newly hatched chicks do walk within several hours (Bekoff, 1976). What are the control parameters underlying these emergent coordinations: hatching, no hatching, walking?

A series of compelling experiments by Bekoff and her colleagues suggest that the pattern generating capability, likely originating early in development, remains intact through all these developmental transitions in behavior, but is modified by sensory input, i.e. the context of the chick. In newly hatched chicks, bending the neck to the right or left, or several other kinds of restraints, restored hatching movements (Bekoff & Kauer, 1982). Indeed, hatching movements could be elicited in chicks up to 61 days of age by folding the birds into appropriately sized glass eggs (Bekoff & Kauer, 1984). Recently Bekoff (1986) demonstrated that modulation EMG burst characteristics in newly hatched chicks are a function of limb loading (i.e., whether the chicks were walking or swimming), again suggesting context-driven output patterns.

In the chick, then, the underlying neural circuitry provides the necessary facilitative substrate, but is not a hard wired prescription for limb coordination. Rather, the specific patterns are emergent with the developmental context. The embryonic posture and/or the constraints of the egg act as the likely control parameters for hatching; perhaps as the chick grows, some critical chick/egg ratio initiates the process. Conversely, we might speculate that upright posture or the sensory consequences of weight bearing shifts the system into locomotor actions of walking or hopping. As in the frog, no neural timer need be invoked to pace these transitions.

Human

Finally, I discuss the effect of birth on the organization of leg movements in humans. Although current ultrasound technology cannot detect the fine elements of intra or interlimb coordination in utero, Prechtl (1986) claims that alternating leg movements appear in human fetuses in the first half of gestation. Heriza (1986) has examined intralimb coordination in low-risk premature infants. She found highly rhythmical and synchronous excursions of hip, knee, and ankle in supine leg kicks in infants ranging from 28 to 36 weeks gestational age and in full-term newborns. The kinematic characteristics of kicks of premature infants and full-term newborns were identical to those described in 2 week to 2 month-old infants

(Thelen & Fisher, 1983). It is likely that in the last months of gestation and the first months of postnatal life, human lower limb movements exhibit a distinct limit cycle attractor regime of considerable stability.

What is the developmental significance of these early coordinated leg movements? Similar to the frog and chick, I believe these actions are manifestations of autonomous pattern generation emergent with the maturity of the neuromotor system. But these movements are neither hard-wired reflexes nor coordinations with function only in the prenatal period (Prechtl, 1986). My colleagues and I have shown that early kicking and stepping is exquisitely context sensitive, especially to conditions which manipulate the mass or load on the legs (Thelen & Fisher, 1982; Thelen, Fisher, & Ridley-Johnson, 1984; Thelen, Fisher, Ridley-Johnson, & Griffin, 1982; Thelen, Skala, & Kelso, 1987). In addition, we have demonstrated the gradual evolution of the pattern generation to a more articulated, complex, and task-appropriate topography (Thelen, 1985; Thelen & Cooke, 1987). Specifically, we believe that the organization of upright locomotion is emergent from the more simple newborn pattern generation with the demands of loading the limbs and maintaining upright posture (Thelen, 1986b). In short, the specific patterns of muscle firings characteristic of mature locomotion grow from the task rather than being imposed upon the task. In this way, the system recruits and modulates the universal tendency to produce patterned output to meet the demands of a complex and changing environment. In humans and in frogs, this adaptation of prenatal spontaneous movement to terrestrial life occurs over a span of many months, while the chick accomplishes the transition in a matter of hours.

One consequence of this view is to direct attention to those aspects of postnatal life that act as potential control parameters in movement production, notably the effects of gravity and those nonneural forces that result when a segmented body moves in space. These have been largely ignored in favor of other neurological and physiological considerations. But a systems view directs us to those non-obvious contributions to developmental change that may indeed have considerable explanatory power, especially in the dramatic transition from the egg or uterine environment to terrestrial existence.

Acknowledgements

I thank Alan Fogel and William Timberlake for their helpful comments on this manuscript. My discussions with J. A. S. Kelso and Alan Fogel were important in formulating these ideas. Carolyn Heriza graciously allowed me to reprint unpublished figures from her dissertation. Preparation of this chapter was supported by National Science Foundation grant BNS 85−09793, NIH grant ROI HD22830, and a Research Career Development Award from NIH.

References

Abraham, R. H., & Shaw, C. D. (1982). *Dynamics—The geometry of behavior.* Santa Cruz, Calif.: Aerial Press.

Bekoff, A. (1976). Ontogeny of leg motor output in the chick embryo: a neural analysis. *Brain Research, 106,* 271−291.

Bekoff, A. (1981). Embryonic development of the neural circuitry underlying motor coordination. In W. M. Cowan (Ed.), *Studies in developmental neurobiology: Essays in honor of Viktor Hamburger,* (pp. 134−170). New York: Oxford University Press.

Bekoff, A. (1986). Is the basic output of the locomotor CPG to flexor and extensor muscles symmetrical? Evidence from walking, swimming, and embryonic motility in chicks. Abstract, Society for Neuroscience Annual Meeting, Washington, D. C. November.

Bekoff, A., & Kauer, J. A. (1982). Neural control of hatching: Role of neck position in turning on hatching movements in post-hatching chicks. *Journal of Comparative Physiology, A, 145,* 497−504.

Bekoff, A., & Kauer, J. A. (1984). Neural control of hatching: Fate of the pattern generator for the leg movements of hatching in post-hatching chicks. *Journal of Neuroscience, 4,* 2659−2666.

Berkinblit, M. B., Feldman, A. G., & Fukson, O. I. (1986). Adaptability of innate motor patterns and motor control mechanisms. *The Behavioral and Brain Sciences, 9,* 585−638.

Fentress, J. C. (1981). Order in ontogeny: Relational dynamics. In K. Immelmann, G. W. Barlow, L. Petrinovitch, & M. Main (Eds.), *Behavioral development: The Bielefeld Interdisciplinary Project,* (pp. 338−371). Cambridge: Cambridge University Press.

Fentress, J. C. (1986). Development of coordinated movement: Dynamic, relational, and multileveled perspectives. In M. G. Wade and H. T. A. Whiting (Eds.), *Motor development in children: Aspects of coordination and control* (pp. 77−105). Dordecht, Netherlands: Martinus Nijhoff Publishers.

Fentress, J. C., & McLeod, P. J. (1986). Motor patterns in development. In E. M. Blass (Ed.), *Handbook of behavioral neurobiology, Vol 8, Developmental psychobiology and developmental neurobiolgy* (pp. 35−97). New York: Plenum.

Fogel, A., & Thelen, E. (1987). The development of expressive and communicative action in the first year: Reinterpreting the evidence from a dynamic systems perspective. *Developmental Psychology, 23,* 747−761.

Haken, H. (1983). *Synergetics: An introduction.* (3rd ed.). Heidelberg: Springer-Verlag.

Haken, H. (Ed.) (1985). *Complex systems: Operational approaches in neurobiology, physics, and computers.* Heidelberg, Berlin: Springer.

Hall, W. G. (1979). Feeding and behavioral activation in infant rats. *Science, 205,* 206−209.

Hall, W. G., & Oppenheim, R. W. (1987). Developmental psychobiology: Prenatal, perinatal, and early postnatal aspects of behavioral development. *Annual Review of Psychology, 38,* 91−128.

Haverkamp, L. (1986). Anatomical and physiological development of the *Xenopus* embryonic motor system in the absence of neural activity. *Journal of Neuroscience, 6,* 1332−1337.

Haverkamp, L., & Oppenheim, R. W. (1986). Behavioral development in the absence of neural activity: Effects of chronic immobilization on amphibian embryos. *Journal of Neuroscience, 6*, 1338−1348.

Heriza, C. (1986). The organization of spontaneous movements in premature infants. Unpublished Ph.D. dissertation, Southern Illinois University.

Kelso, J. A. S., & Scholz, J. P. (1985). Cooperative phenomena in biological motion. In H. Haken (Ed.), *Synergetics of complex systems in physics, chemistry, and biology*, (pp. 124−149) New York: Springer-Verlag.

Kelso, J. A. S., Scholz, J. P., & Schöner, G. (1986). Non-equilibrium phase transitions in coordinated biological motion: Critical fluctuations. *Physics Letters A, 118*, 279−284.

Kelso, J. A. S., & Schöner, G. (1987). Toward a physical (synergetic) theory of biological coordination. In R. Graham (Ed.), *Lasers and synergetics, Springer Proceeding in Physics Vol. 19* (pp. 224−237). Heidelberg, Berlin: Springer.

Kugler, P. N., Kelso, J. A. S., & Turvey, M. T. (1980). On the concept of coordinative structures as dissipative structures. I. Theoretical lines of convergence. In G. E. Stelmach & J. Requin (Eds.), *Tutorials in motor behavior* (pp. 3−47). New York: North Holland.

Kugler, P., Kelso, J. A. S., & Turvey, M. T. (1982). On the control and co-ordination of naturally developing systems. In J. A. S. Kelso & J. E. Clark (Eds.), *The development of movement control and co-oordination* (pp. 5−78). New York: John Wiley.

Nicolis, J. S. (1986). *Dynamics of hierarchical systems: An evolutionary approach.* Berlin: Springer-Verlag.

Okamoto, T. & Goto, Y. (1985). Human infant pre-independent and independent walking. In S. Kondo (Ed.), *Primate morphophysiology, locomotor analyses and human bipedalism* (pp. 25−45). Tokyo, Japan: University of Tokyo Press.

Oppenheim, R. W., Pittman, R., Gray, M., & Maderdrut, J. L. (1978) Embryonic behavior, hatching, and neuromuscular development in the chick following a transient reduction of spontaneous motility and sensory input by neuromuscular blocking agents. *Journal of Comparative Neurology, 179*, 619−640.

Oyama, S. (1985). *The ontogeny of information: Developmental systems and evolution.* Cambridge: Cambridge University Press.

Prechtl, H. F. R. (1981). The study of neural development as a perspective of clinical problems. In K. J. Connolly & H. F. R. Prechtl (Eds.), *Maturation and development: Biological and psychological perspectives*, (pp. 198−215). London: Spastics International and William Heinemann.

Prechtl, H. F. R. (1986). Prenatal motor development. In M. G. Wade and H. T. A. Whiting (Eds.), *Motor development in children: Aspects of coordination and control* (pp. 53−64). Dordecht, Netherlands: Martinus Nijhoff Publishers.

Provine, R. R. (1981). Development of wing-flapping and flight in normal and flap-deprived domestic chicks. *Developmental Psychobiology, 14*, 279−291.

Provine, R. R. (1986). Behavioral neuroembryology: Motor perspectives. In W. T. Greenough & J. M. Juraska (Eds.), *Developmental neuropsychobiology* (pp. 213−239). New York: Academic Press.

Robertson, S. S., Dierker, L. J., Sorokin, Y., & Rosen, M. G. (1982). Human fetal movement: Spontaneous oscillations near one cycle per minute. *Science, 218*, 1327−1330.

Robinson, S. R., & Smotherman, W. P. (1987). Environmental determinants of behaviour in the rat fetus. II. The emergence of synchronous movement. *Animal Behaviour, 35*, 1652−1662.

Schöner, G., Haken, H., & Kelso, J. A. S. (1986). A stochastic theory of phase transitions in human hand movement. *Biological Cybernetics, 53*, 1−11.

Smotherman, W. P., & Robinson, S. R. (1988). The uterus as environment: The ecology of fetal experience. In E. M. Blass (Ed.), *Handbook of behavioral neurobiology, Vol. 9, Developmental psychobiology behavioral ecology*, (pp. 149–196). New York: Plenum.

Stehouwer, D. J., & Farel, P. B. (1983). Development of hindlimb locomotor activity in the bullfrog (*Rana catesbeiana*) studied in vitro. *Science, 219*, 516–518.

Stehouwer, D. J., & Farel, P. B. (1984). Development of hindlimb locomotor behavior in the frog. *Developmental Psychobiology, 17*, 217–232.

Stehouwer, D. J., & Farel, P. B. (1985). Development of locomotor mechanisms in the frog. *Journal of Neurophysiology, 53*, 1453–1466.

Thelen, E. (1985). Developmental origins of motor coordination: Leg movements in human infants. *Developmental Psychobiology, 18*, 1–22.

Thelen, E. (1986a). Treadmill-elicited stepping in seven-month-old infants. *Child Development, 57*, 1498–1506.

Thelen, E. (1986b). Development of coordinated movement: implications for early human development. In M. G. Wade & H. T. A. Whiting (Eds.), *Motor skills acquisition* (pp. 107–124). Dordecht (Netherlands): Martinus Nijhoff Publishers.

Thelen, E. and Cooke, D. W. (1987). The relationship between newborn stepping and later locomotion: A new interpretation. *Developmental Medicine and Child Neurology, 29*, 380–393.

Thelen, E., & Fisher, D. M. (1982). Newborn stepping: An explanation for a "disappearing reflex." *Developmental Psychology, 18*, 760–775.

Thelen, E., & Fisher, D. M. (1983). The organization of spontaneous leg movements in newborn infants. *Journal of Motor Behavior, 15*, 353–377.

Thelen, E., Fisher, D. M., & Ridley-Johnson, R. (1984). The relationship between physical growth and a newborn reflex. *Infant Behavior and Development, 7*, 479–493.

Thelen, E., Fisher, D. M., Ridley-Johnson, R., & Griffin, N. (1982). The effects of body build and arousal on newborn infant stepping. *Developmental Psychobiology, 15*, 447–453.

Thelen, E., & Fogel, A. (in press). Toward an action-based theory of infant development. In J. Lockman & N. Hazen (Eds.), *Action in social context*, New York: Plenum.

Thelen, E., Kelso, J. A. S., & Fogel, A. (1987). Self-organizing systems and infant motor development. *Developmental Review, 7*, 39–65.

Thelen, E., Skala, K., & Kelso, J. A. S. (1987). The dynamic nature of early coordination: Evidence from bilateral leg movements in young infants. *Developmental Psychology, 23*, 179–186.

Wolff, P. H. (1986). The maturation and development of fetal motor patterns. In M. G. Wade & H. T. A. Whiting (Eds.), *Motor skills acquisition*, (pp. 65–74). Dordecht (Netherlands): Martinus Nijhoff Publishers.

CLOSING COMMENTARY

On Fetal Development: A Behavioral Perspective

Norman A. Krasnegor

Human Learning and Behavior Branch
National Institute of Child Health and Human Development
National Institutes of Health
Bethesda, Maryland

During the past decade, psychobiologists have evidenced a heightened interest in and research on that aspect of ontogeny known as the perinatal period (Krasnegor, 1987a). This phase of development includes the time span that, in the human infant, extends from the seventh month of gestation to the completion of the first month after birth. Experimental studies conducted during this phase have great promise because they provide the potential for viewing the emergence of essential biological and behavioral processes necessary for normal development to proceed on course (Krasnegor, in press).

Of equal importance to this trend in psychobiological research is that which has been observed in the field of neonatology (Krasnegor, 1987a). This subdivision of biomedicine, established some 25 years ago, focuses upon the study and care of babies born at risk, due in large part to premature birth, intrauterine growth retardation (IUGR) or developmental disabilities. To deal with these ill babies, neonatolologists established the neonatal intensive care unit (NICU). This specialized environment comprises a highly skilled staff of nurses and physicians who employ uniquely designed instrumentation to diagnose and treat these tiny (less than 2500 g) immature humans. While great progress has been made during the last quarter century in reducing the morbidity and mortality of these babies, a recognition has gradually emerged that further improvement in outcome requires a multidisciplinary approach. This implies the acquisition of knowledge concerning both behavioral and biological development that occurs during the perinatal period (Krasnegor, 1987a). It is clear that during this period there is a dynamic interplay between a baby's biological heritage and its behavior that is necessary for achieving a successful adaptation to its new environment outside of the womb.

Recently, neonatologists have developed the technical capability to routinely care for and sustain the viability of babies weighing only 1500 g.

They have even begun to admit and treat in the NICU babies weighing as little as 500—750 g. But for the fact that these tiny humans were "born", they are for all intents and purposes equivalent to the fetus still developing in the womb. If these babies can be successfully managed and maintained from a biological point of view, what will be the quality of their lives as they develop? The answer to this question, in part, relates to whether a deep understanding of their behavior can be achieved. Successful attainment of this goal should allow the knowledge gained to be applied to the task of fostering an appropriate behavioral repertoire, which can maximize the likelihood of normal development.

Of course, research of the type suggested cannot be carried out on sick babies, particularly ones which are are so fragile and hover between life and death. But the need for basic knowledge of behavior during this early phase of development still exists. That is why psychobiological research on perinatal animals, both extant and planned, is so important. While it can be argued that such basic research is motivated by the quest for new knowledge and discovery of the unknown, the work described in this volume relates directly to knowledge gaps alluded to above. The new findings and ideas derived from behavioral research on nonhuman mammalian fetuses can provide basic information for clinicians to craft treatment strategies and principles to redesign the treatment environment. When viewed from this perspective, basic research on behavioral development of the fetus relates logically to a rationale of high purpose and great potential benefit.

CHARACTERIZATION OF BEHAVIOR

How is fetal behavior to be characterized? One might consider at least three possible ways. These lie along a continuum that can be described in the following way. At one extreme lies the "top-down" approach to definition and analysis. This approach describes behavior in terms of higher level processes, such as perception or cognition, that in effect refer to a "conceptual nervous system". In this system, the behavior of the fetus is viewed as an epiphenomenon that is useful to the extent that it reveals and informs about high-level neural processes. At the other end of the continuum lies the "bottom-up" or molecular approach for characterizing and analyzing behavior. Single cells or groups of neurons are studied and models are derived based on their patterns of interaction. Behavior in such an analytic system is conceived of as specific patterns of neural output from assemblages of elements that are organized during ontogenesis.

In the middle lies a descriptive, empirical approach to characterizing behavior. This approach relies on systematic observations of what an intact organism does by cataloguing frequency and duration of particular acts over a specified period of ontogeny. No reference is made to higher-level or molecular processes in defining behavior. These observations serve to provide a baseline of normative development against which a functional analysis of behavior can be carried out. The middle course, exemplified in the work of Smotherman and Robinson (this volume), raises the question of how the frequency, duration and organization of behavior changes over the course of gestation. Smotherman and Robinson have demonstrated methods for characterizing the ontogenetic organization of movement and experimentally manipulating the intrauterine environment to assess fetal capacity for simple learning. More research along these lines by additional investigators can provide a bridge between the top-down and bottom-up approaches to the study of perinatal behavioral development. Representative examples of each of these approaches can be found in this volume.

The observational study of fetal behavior raises another important question: Which behaviors in the fetal repertoire are necessary and sufficient to allow fetal development to proceed normally? This query may be answered, in part, by discerning two categories of behavior. The first of these includes endogenous behaviors which are sufficient for the completion of the in-utero phase of development (ontogenetic adaptation). The second includes behaviors that are necessary for the organism to adapt to the postnatal environment (preparation).

BEHAVIORAL CAPACITY DURING FETAL DEVELOPMENT

Besides posing questions concerning the endogenous behavioral patterns of the fetus extant during gestation, researchers also have conducted functional analyses of the fetus's capacity to behave. The work reported includes non-invasive studies of human fetuses at approximately the same developmental stage. Studies of learning and memory, auditory perception, and circadian rhythms have been undertaken.

The work on learning (Kolata, 1984; Krasnegor, in press, see also Smotherman & Robinson this volume) has clearly documented that the fetal rat pup is capable of associative conditioning during gestation. These findings help to pinpoint when central nervous system anatomical organization is sufficient to functionally subsume the type of conditioning investigated. This work also demonstrates that learning in-utero can be retained for over two weeks postnatally. This important finding indicates the fetal capacity for memory of learned associations. The results raise the interesting questions of whether associative conditioning is a basic mechanism employed by the fetus to encode sensory information and whether information acquired prenatally can be used to adapt the fetus to its postnatal environment.

Anatomical and acoustical studies have clearly established that, in the last trimester, the human fetal auditory system is sufficiently developed to analyze sound stimuli. Moreover, recordings taken from within the birth canal just prior to delivery demonstrate that maternal voice can easily be heard by the developing fetus. This conclusion has been confirmed by studies which demonstrate that neonates recognize their mother's voice on the first day of life and discriminate auditory stimuli that were presented to them during gestation (see Fifer & Moon, this volume).

Work on analyzing the circadian rhythms of rat fetuses indicates that they are in phase with the external environment (see Reppert & Weaver, this volume). The studies carried out point to the mother as the mediator that programs the fetal circadian clock. This implies that the capacity for synchronization with the light/dark cycle exists prior to birth. This aspect of the fetal repertoire is clearly one that prepares pups for adaptation to the postnatal environment.

These examples attest to the wide range of behavioral capacities that human and rat fetuses possess. They also are indicative of what remains to be discovered. The work of Fifer and his colleagues is particularly instructive. The findings on maternal voice recognition derived from normal children are being extended to premature infants. This research is an excellent example of the raison d'etre for investigating fetal behavioral development as outlined above. By understanding the development of voice recognition in the normal fetus, one can begin to address the problems of behavioral deficiencies observed in the premature infant. This should aid neonatologists in devising more effective treatment for their patients based on the knowledge of whether they can recognize and thus become appropriately attached to their mother.

CONCLUSION

The publication of this volume attests to the recognition that a new frontier of developmental psychobiology has been identified and is under active research (Krasnegor, 1987b). The quest that motivates the ideas described herein relates to the creative search for answers to the unknown and to gain access to the data which form an essential aspect of behavioral development. This pursuit after new knowledge will complement the needs identified by neonatologists, who are themselves approaching a threshold in clinical care of the premature infant.

References

Kolata, G. (1984). Studying learning in the womb. *Science, 225*, 302−303.

Krasnegor, N.A. (1987a). Introduction. In N. A. Krasnegor, E. M. Blass, M. A. Hofer & W. P. Smotherman, (Eds.), *Perinatal Development: A Psychobiological Perspective*, (pp. 1−8). Orlando: Academic Press.

Krasnegor, N. A. (1987b). Developmental psychobiology research: A health scientist administrator's perspective. *Developmental Psychobiology, 20*, 641−644.

Krasnegor, N. A. (in press). Measurement of learning, sensory and linquistic capacity early in life: a selective overview of recent research. In A. Galaburda, (Ed.), *From Neurons to Dyslexia*. Cambridge: MIT Press.